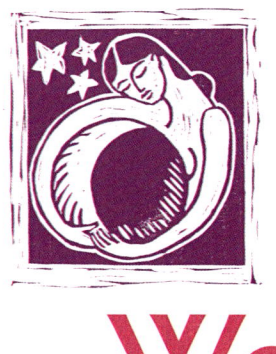

The Woman's Quest

...unfolding women's path of power and wisdom

A 13-session course

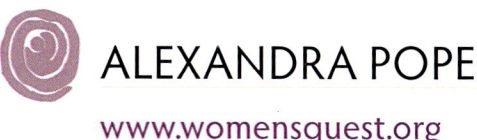

ALEXANDRA POPE

www.womensquest.org

© Alexandra Pope 2006 · Updated 2009 and 2013 · All rights reserved

The Woman's Quest

....

A Bright Pen Book

Copyright © Alexandra Pope 2013

Cover and layout by Toni Lumsden ©

All rights reserved. No part of this publication may be reproduced, stored in a retrieval system, or transmitted in any form or by any means, electronic, mechanical, photocopy, recording or otherwise, without prior written permission of the copyright owner. Nor can it be circulated in any form of binding or cover other than that in which it is published and without similar condition including this condition being imposed on a subsequent purchaser.

British Library Cataloguing Publication Data.

A catalogue record for this book is available from the British Library

ISBN 978-0-7552-1564-5

Authors OnLine Ltd
19 The Cinques
Gamlingay, Sandy
Bedfordshire SG19 3NU
England

This book is also available in e-book format, details of which are available at www.authorsonline.co.uk

....

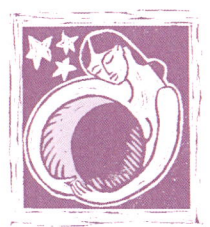

Contents

Introduction		4
Getting started		8
Initiating your power		10
Session 1:	Getting to know your cycle	16
Session 2:	Mapping the four phases of the cycle	18
Session 3:	Inner work and the premenstruum	21
Session 4:	Losing it, using it – power and the premenstruum	24
Session 5:	Power and the critic	26
Session 6:	The bitch – your inner power broker	30
Session 7:	Power and vulnerability	32
Session 8:	Liminality and creativity	34
Session 9:	Intuition, guidance and meaning making	37
Session 10:	Intimacy and relationship	40
Session 11:	Initiation, ecstasy and shamanism	43
Session 12:	Time, timeliness and timing	46
Session 13:	Embodying your wisdom	48
Epilogue:	Women are blessed	51
Appendix:	Menarche Ritual	52
Menstrual dreaming charts		55
Acknowledgements		58

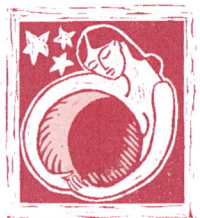

Introduction

THE WOMAN'S QUEST FOR POWER AND WISDOM

Centered in a uniquely female process – the menstrual cycle – and using practices and principles affirming to women, **The Woman's Quest** is an intelligent and creative 13-menstrual months spiritual guide, grounded in female ways. A self-development programme for women, **The Woman's Quest** takes you on a journey of discovery and recovery, of power and wisdom gathering. Embodying cyclical consciousness and the power of the feminine, you can come to know a deeper sense of love, empowerment and healing. It's a journey in which the individual and the world are intimately interwoven.

WHY PAY ATTENTION TO THE CYCLE?

As women we have an enormous elemental intelligence that informs our emotional and spiritual development. The menstrual cycle is like the yoga or Tao of women – a template for psychological and spiritual evolution, an innate intelligence that works, guides and matures you. A repeating rhythm you can't control, the cycle is your training ground for coming to know and love this elemental intelligence. It is the menstrual cycle itself that creates the tension necessary for you to fully embody this elemental presence.

The cycle is an organic process of timing that is uncontrolled by the inorganic societal timing imposed from outside. An inner referencing guide, it can initiate you into deep altered states, cultivating your authority and wisdom. The years of menstruating give you the compound interest from each monthly process, your body inducting you into something larger and larger. Then, when you arrive at the door of menopause, you will have some inkling of the nature of this transition and be able to reap the full harvest of its challenges and riches.

The talents of your cycle are to some extent a given. However, to be able to access the fullness of what is available you need to pay deep attention to the process and be willing to follow it.

THE MENSTRUAL CYCLE:

- Cultivates emotional and spiritual intelligence
- Builds inner authority
- Facilitates a deeper intimacy with self and union with another
- Develops interdependent consciousness
- Deepens appreciation of meaning and purpose in life
- Strengthens intuitive and psychic ability
- Awakens the activist in us
- Teaches us about the dynamics of the creative process
- Educates us in the art of understanding energy and timing
- Initiates (along with the transitions of menarche, pregnancy and birth and menopause).
- Is a crucial preparation of embodiment for the process of pregnancy and birth
- Is a natural healing system

MENSTRUATION IS:

- An altered state of consciousness
- A natural visionary state
- The grace of renewal and inspiration
- A moment of connection with ones deepest or highest self, with the World.

MANIFESTING YOUR DREAMS

By developing tools to create and sustain a meaningful and rich life through knowledge of the cycle, you'll discover your own Menstrual Dreaming. The wisdom of menstruation, menstrual dreaming is the deep intelligence of female embodied existence. Through the stories, or dreaming, your body reveals your spirituality and power, your calling and connection to the world. It is your ally in manifesting your goals and life calling.

YOUR PERSONAL QUEST

This 13-session course takes you on a quest to discover:

- How to access the wise power of female embodied life
- The means for manifesting your calling and maturing a deep inner authority
- How to open doors to ecstatic states and a woman's natural vision questing time
- The different creative phases of the menstrual cycle and how to get the most out of them
- Your natural times of heightened inspiration and wisdom gathering
- Your times for activity and your times for dreaming
- How to strengthen self-care and, for those who suffer from menstrual problems, healing
- How to become your own life coach through knowledge of the cycle
- 13 indispensable allies for the woman's path
- The truth about the menstrual story
- The power of the Feminine
- A stronger sense of belonging in and care of the World.

WHAT YOU WILL EXPLORE

Spread over 13 menstrual monthly sessions to give you time to mature into the process and for the magic of time to work on you, each session can be its own self-contained learning/discovery/initiatory experience. It is an opening to a specific topic that will deepen over time.

Month 1:	Getting to know the cycle
Month 2:	Mapping the cycle
Month 3:	Inner work and the premenstruum
Month 4:	Losing it, using it – power and the premenstruum
Month 5:	Power and the critic
Month 6:	The bitch – your inner power broker
Month 7:	Power and vulnerability
Month 8:	Liminality and creativity
Month 9:	Intuition, guidance and meaning making
Month 10:	Intimacy and relationship
Month 11:	Initiation, ecstasy and shamanism
Month 12:	Time, timeliness and timing
Month 13:	Embodying your wisdom

IS THE COURSE REALLY FOR ME?

If you're in your menstruating years and are interested in **leadership**, **creativity**, **spirituality**, **wellbeing**, **counselling** and **psychotherapy**, **coaching**, **change**, **activism/world work**, **shamanism**, and the **work of Soul**, this course is the right choice. Regardless of how busy you are you can do this course. While there is some time commitment involved, the main commitment is a readiness to question previous beliefs and ways of doing things. Although it's not a quick fix, you might be surprised at how quickly the 'gold' appears once you start making changes. You'll be using a different kind of consciousness – modes of being and acting that refuse to be motivated, forced or bullied into action. It's about a deep allowing through which emerges an enormous elemental intelligence that can guide, motivate and anoint your life with an enormous grace.

WHAT IF MY CYCLE IS IRREGULAR?

I encourage you to follow the rhythm that is your cycle, however strange and erratic it may seem. This may mean the course takes longer to complete. If the gaps between periods are very long, you might want to read ahead to other sessions and find ways to combine them.

You might also want to try doing the **Deer Exercise** (a Taoist practice that involves a self massage and breathing process that takes about 5 –10 minutes each day to do). This exercise is a marvellous practice for healing menstrual problems and regulating the cycle. You will find a description of how to do the exercise in my co-authored book *The Pill: are you sure it's for you* (Allen and Unwin, 2008)

WHAT IF I'M ON THE PILL?

This presents a dilemma because, apart from the mini pill, all others interrupt the cycle and, even if you give yourself monthly 'bleeds' this is not like a normal menstrual bleed and the cycle is not a normal cycle. The mini pill, rather than interrupting the cycle, affects the lining of the womb so that it becomes a hostile environment for implantation, as well as keeping the mucous infertile. Some women do experience mood changes on the Pill that are similar to the classic premenstrual ones leading up to the monthly 'bleed.' This I cannot explain except to say that it is as if the spirit of the real cycle cannot be silenced and tries to speak anyway. The Pill also has a flattening effect on your feelings and cuts you off from your depths. To reap the full rewards of this course you would need to be off the Pill.

If you use the Pill for contraceptive purposes, do check out *The Contraception Kit* by Francesca Naish and Jane Bennett, **www.nfmcontraception.com**
If you take the Pill for health reasons, consider working with a holistic health practitioner, as there are many natural ways for easing and healing menstrual problems. Check out my books *The Wild Genie: the Healing Power of Menstruation*, *Walking with the Genie: the Modern Woman's Menstrual Health Kit*, or *The Pill: are you sure it's for you?* (co-authored with Jane Bennett) in which we also address how to heal menstrual problems.

WILL I HAVE TO CHANGE MY DIET?

Throughout the course I will suggest health tips, such as dietary suggestions, for you to try. Your physical wellbeing is not separate from your psychological and spiritual wellbeing. In fact much premenstrual moodiness can be significantly eased with a great diet. Feeling nourished also makes it easier to expand into, and handle, the heightened states of menstruation. If you suffer from extreme menstrual problems, this course will be a vital step in healing them, and may even prove revelatory to you.

WHAT ABOUT DRUGS?

If you are dependent on drugs (legal and illegal), alcohol, cigarettes, caffeine or sugar they will affect your experience of the cycle and the degree of depth you may access. The irony is that if you're using these substances heavily it may be that you are psychologically highly sensitive already but you don't yet know how to live into it for whatever reason. Some of you may enjoy the above on an occasional basis. During the course I will suggest that you go without, particularly leading into and during bleeding. Menstruation itself is already an altered state of consciousness, and to take a mood altering substance during that time can both aggravate and blunt the natural experience.

DOES IT MATTER IF I MISS A MONTH OF DOING THE COURSE?

Even with the best will in the world life intervenes and you find a month has slipped by and you've barely attended to the Quest. That can happen. And it's fine; simply pick up where you left off. You might find you can combine two sessions into one month if you're getting the hang of the process. Don't let it derail you forever. Just do the best you can within the circumstances you find yourself. You are learning a practice; a way of being that is with you for life and not just the 13 'months' of the course. Some women are working with the **Woman's Quest** in groups. This is an ideal way to sustain the program and possibly access greater depth and meaning.

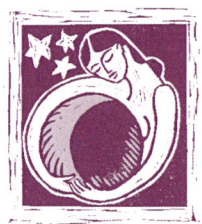

Getting started

TOOLS

You will need the following to do the **Woman's Quest**:

- Your **Woman's Quest journal** – a journal devoted purely to this course. Buy, create or decorate one that feels good to you.

- The **Menstrual Dreaming** chart. You will find this on page 55. Make copies of it and keep the original for the purposes of copying. You will need one for each month for a while (possibly more if your cycle is very long). As the chart is only A4 size, I recommend you enlarge this to A3 when you photocopy it. For those who find A3 still too small to work with, create something that feels more appropriate for your needs or simply use your journal.

SESSION GUIDANCE

- When I speak of 'month' I am referring to the menstrual month. Day one of the 'month' is the first day of bleeding (this does not include spotting). A session refers to a month of your cycle.

- Each session builds on the previous one; it will be like adding another layer each month.

- Each session has a **focus**, which contains introductory information for the particular topic of that session, followed by **What You Need to Do** including exercises/practices and questions to guide and deepen you into the topic. The questions are merely to get your creative juices flowing for reflection in your journal. You don't have to answer them all. Equally you can make up your own. **What You Need To Do** has at least two steps. Step 1 is a self-care activity and the following steps are related to the topic of that session. Some sessions are lengthier than others.

- Engage with each session at the beginning of each cycle and set your intention for the coming month. Particularly in the early phases of the Quest aim, as best you can, to have a check-in moment each day to fill in the Menstrual Dreaming chart or reflect in your journal on some of the questions asked in each session.

- If your cycle is reasonably regular it might help to also mark in your diary key times for you to pay special attention for specific things, for example when you are entering your most creative, energised, vulnerable or difficult moments, and either capitalise on or care for such moments. With time you won't need to do that because you will feel it so intrinsically, although always noting roughly when you think menstruation is due is usually wise to do.

- Throughout I refer to the word 'world' with both a small 'w' and capital 'W'. When I use 'world' I am referring to the material world we deal with every day – the physical, familial, social, economic and political worlds. When I refer to the World I am speaking of something beyond the mundane, of spiritual realities – World as spiritual presence, a co-creating force, a symbol of divine forces, as something sacred that envelops the mundane world.

- Your feelings about and experience of menstruation are sometimes connected with what happened to you when you first menstruated. Some of you may have got off to a rather negative, uninspired or downright bad start. Fortunately all is not lost. Through ritual you can re-imagine and reset the beginning of the journey into womanhood. I have included a special ritual for this purpose in the appendix. I recommend you do this ritual at some point during the course. It's ideal to do it with one other person but, if that's not possible, do it on your own.

> **COACHING**
>
> The **Woman's Quest** is designed to stand-alone. You can however add another level of richness with coaching. This will help you to keep the focus and also open up new avenues of awareness and depth of feeling. The added input will make the process more potent. For coaching do get in touch with me on:
>
> Mob: **+44 07974 388 973** or email: **info@womensquest.org**

A LITTLE DREAMING BEFORE YOU START

Before you embark on the course give some thought to the following:

- List those areas of your life for which you seek guidance. They might be places of confusion, uncertainty, anxiety or inaction/stagnation.
- What do you want to achieve or discover? (This question applies to both current and longer-term intentions, as well as deeper issues of meaning and overall life direction, the spiritual and the mundane).
- What do you hope to get from doing the course?
- Write the responses in your journal, leaving a blank page or two to come back and add extra ideas as they come to you. Aim to refine the list to come up with a few key themes, goals or issues that feel the most important. Read them out loud as though you were declaring them to an audience. Your audience in this case is the universe.

"My intentions are to..."

"The issues that I'm seeking clarification and direction on are..."

(*This is only a suggestion; find a wording that works for you*)

Now that you have done that you can put it to one side. The first month of the course is a gentle entry. Don't try to be too focused on goals. This doesn't mean that you forget or abandon them but what you will do is drop the 'trying to find the answers/solutions' mode of being. Neither does it mean sit on your bum and do nothing. Just have them quietly resting inside you. If you like you can create an image of them through drawing or montage of images (include a photo of yourself in the collage) so they are held in another way. I want you to imagine that the guidance you seek and the means to realise your ambitions might actually be seeking you.

Now you are ready to be initiated into the Quest. The next chapter 'Initiating Your Power' prepares you psychologically for the course. Don't be tempted to skip it, as you will get some important guidance.

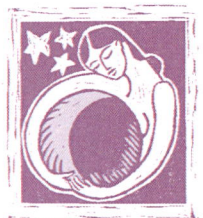

Initiating your power

Women have been taught to deny, distrust, despise and dismiss a wonderful force in our bodies, even treating it as a momentary insanity making us essentially unstable and feeling full of shame. In modern times there has been an attempt to clean up this negativity by treating the menstrual cycle as a purely biological process. But in reducing it to merely a physiological function we have stripped it of its deeper meanings and experiences – its ability to open us to deep soul forces, to altered states, and our psycho-spiritual template. Within all that historical negativity and darkness lies a story of power that has been denied. We are still denying that force today.

Our failure to address the cycle as a truly empowering, mystical process, I believe, contributes to low self-esteem, depression, anxiety, eating disorders, body image problems, addictions, relationship conflicts as well as menstrual and menopausal problems. It deprives women of a wonderful source of wisdom, creativity and renewal – an ally for negotiating life.

I believe women are now fed a spiritual and personal development language that may have more to do with men than women. We have our own amazing inner teacher, guide, initiator and 'practice' for psychological and spiritual evolution, yet these days tend to seek it on the outside with methods that are more relevant to men. In failing to value female ways, a violence is perpetrated.

AN ENORMOUS ELEMENTAL FORCE

There is an enormous elemental force at work in women's bodies that is both intensely intimate and universal – ecstatic, creative, restorative and full of love. We experience this force at menstruation (and also during pregnancy and giving birth). The post-menopausal woman, who has understood and lived the journey of the cycle, fully inhabits this power.

This ecstatic experience does not have to be struggled or sweated for, or heroically earned. If we are willing to court the life of our bodies we are given privileged access to something Other that happens naturally without the techniques we normally employ such as meditation, prayer, yoga, fasting, sweat lodges, vision quests, drugs and so on. The monthly round of the menstrual cycle itself is our means of induction or initiation into this energy. It acts as a kind of training ground to reap the fullness of what is a natural gift to us – an alchemical vessel within which we individuate. And menstruation itself is alchemical.

The process of the cycle also prepares a woman for the psychological and spiritual challenges of pregnancy, birth and menopause, which are all in their own right, powerful states of consciousness. At its most basic level, the cycle is the stress sensitive, and therefore inner guidance system, in women. A woman in touch with her cycle and using it as a feedback system, is practising preventative medicine, experiencing her own natural in built de-stressing and self soothing system, creating a more fulsome intelligence, and working much more effectively. Awareness of the cycle is vitalising, creating a feeling of specialness and sweet intimacy. This is healing and empowering. It is a blessing.

THE RECOVERY OF THE SACRED AND THE FEMALE BODY

The body is a source of the sacred. Patriarchal religion has everywhere denied this fact and the female body has copped the lion's share of that denial. There has been and still is to some extent a deep loathing and opprobrium towards the female body, which women have absorbed. Spiritual life is impoverished without the deeply desirous, sensuous nature of our bodies. Our bodies are the gateway to the Ecstatic or the Sacred Feminine. We cannot have ecstasy without our flesh and blood nature. Beauty, love, tenderness and joy blossom in the vulnerability that is known as we fully enter the life of the body. And in women, the menstrual cycle enhances that process.

UNDERSTANDING POWER

There are three kinds of power – power over, power with and power from within. *Power over* is your capacity to shape and manipulate your world/environment, to impose your will. This is Mastery. *Power with* is your capacity for engagement with what is – to cooperate, co-create, to be touched and to touch, to allow the unknown to speak and guide you. This is Mystery. *Power from within* is about your inner authority, your inner wisdom or intelligence and the vitality that that generates. It comes from making greater peace with yourself, and experiencing a sense of oneness. This is Empowerment. You are cultivating all these expressions of power through the dynamic of the cycle; you are moving beyond mastery to artistry. Power grows as you learn how to hold and channel the elemental, ecstatic forces of your being, handling the tension of the conflicting currents of consciousness and learning how to ride the currents as you shift from one consciousness to the other.[1]

---

[1] Thanks to Starhawk for the idea of the 3 types of power from her book *Dreaming the Dark,* Unwin Hyman Ltd, London, 1990. The elucidation of the three types is largely my own.

What is the power of the cycle?

- Power is the elemental, ecstatic force unleashed at menstruation
- Power is the experiencing of deep oneness at menstruation
- Power is the wisdom that matures in us through the monthly cycling
- Power is coming to know and love oneself
- Power is the embodying of the Deep Feminine
- Power is feeling the presence of Grace, of being touched by that which is abiding.
- Power is intimacy
- Power is the act of awareness
- Power is surrender
- Power is the capacity to enter into and hold the tension of the 'not known' for the new creative possibilities to emerge
- Power is being able to assert oneself
- Power is the capacity to take charge of ones life and realise ones goals.

HOW DO YOU GET IN TOUCH WITH THE POWER OF THE CYCLE?

Getting in touch with the power of menstruation mainly comes from what you don't do. It is the technique-less way. The secret blessings of menstruation, of your innate authority, do not have to be struggled for, or heroically earned. Instead you must face into the experience, obverse and embody and above all let yourself be moved.

If you are willing to court the rhythmical life of your body you are given access to something Other that happens naturally. And the very act of courting the inner life of your body itself builds an inner sweetness, surety and dignity – a spirit of sovereign authority that is priceless.

THERE ARE FOUR KEY ELEMENTS TO UNFOLDING YOUR INNER RICHES:

- *Pay attention* through charting the cycle, writing a journal, recording your dreams, taking time.
- Practice in some measure *the thirteen allies* (the thirteen S's) of the technique-less way: silence, solitude, stillness, surrender, simplicity, slowness, softness, self-interest, serenity, sanctuary, sacred, support, sleep. (This list grew over numerous workshops. It was a delightful serendipity that each word began with an S).
- *Hold the charge* by staying close to your inner experience and sustaining the tension of the shifting currents of consciousness.
- *Value yourself* by having the courage to believe in your process, follow it and be called to account where necessary.

PAY ATTENTION

A deep process of awareness, the first task is to get to know your cycle. (Session 1 and 2 will guide you in how to do this.) Awareness of the cycle is an ongoing project. It's empowering just to know where you are in the cycle at any moment – to sense ovulation, to feel the shift of mood and feeling as you get closer to menstruation, to recognize the pattern of your dream life and all the other signs and signals. By charting your cycle, you are building a deep self-acceptance of and a wonderful quiet intimacy with yourself. Over time this growing acceptance and intimacy strengthens your capacity to hold the charge and depth that you are gifted with at menstruation. Without this inner capacity, which is like an inner container, the charge can be disruptive, wasted and lost. When this happens we miss an opportunity for psycho-spiritual evolution and can end up having the mother of all reckonings at menopause.

PRACTICE THE THIRTEEN ALLIES

Allow yourself a dose of the thirteen allies – silence, solitude, stillness, surrender, simplicity, slowness, softness, self-interest, serenity, sanctuary, sacred, support and sleep – however small, as you come into and during menstruation. (I will suggest ones to focus on for each session)

Ideally it would be wonderful to be able to shut up shop for at least a day of delicious time out and rest without having to attend to anyone else. However, the demands of 21st century life seem to work against such pleasures. Fortunately our psyches appear to be remarkably long suffering. If you can give at least some gesture in the direction of your inner life and needs at menstruation through the practice of the allies that is still a plus and means something to your deep self. It also builds a new habit, or practice, that will be easier to do next time round. You may not be able to take a whole day off but it could be one evening. It may be that you don't cook dinner that night and your partner does. For an incredibly busy mother it might mean sitting down with a cup of tea for half an hour and absolutely saying "no" to everything and everyone for that time. It may mean simply doing something different. To do something different once is to irrevocably shift the axis of things. It does mean doing something that feels nourishing to your whole being and not something that just feels like a good idea. You may not be able to do it on the first day of your period but if your day off is the day before, or on day 2 or 3 of the cycle, I've noticed it still seems to work for the psyche and the body to some extent. Be inventive. Above all claim the right to have time just for you.

The Thirteen Allies

Silence: Take some time without TV (especially have a news fast), music, computers, mobiles etc. Go into a cone of silence and let the zone of menstruation claim you.

Solitude: Make sure you get genuine empty space for yourself where you're not in relating mode.

Stillness: Hang out, potter (this can create a lovely inner stillness), lie down, do nothing, stare into space, just find someway to STOP mentally as well as physically.

Surrender: Drop your endless agendas, aspirations and ambitions and momentarily 'die' (check out 'stillness').

Simplicity: Just do the basics of daily living now, no complicated cooking for family or organising some great project. Keep it simple.

Slowness: This means moving at the actual pace of your being and not everyone else's timing. You may feel considerably slowed down, but don't be fooled for one minute into thinking that you're somehow less capable or productive. Actually you're profoundly connected to yourself – now *that's* power.

Softness: Practice genuine tenderness and generosity with yourself. No tough regimes. Although these might be good or necessary to have, in this moment they work against the exquisite subtlety and intimacy that is possible at menstruation.

Self-interest: Practice undiluted self-interest. And no, it's not selfishness; it's self-interestedness and self-preservation. Others indeed may not like it but, remember, that could be their own apparent selfishness speaking. This is truly the time when you unashamedly give to yourself.

Serenity: Cruise, glide, keep a certain detachment from the stuff of the world, even if it looks momentarily about to collapse, maintain a certain serene bubble of detachment about you.

Sanctuary: Create a feeling of specialness or sanctuary by having a sense of order in your physical environment, even if it's just your bedroom. Often women do have a frenzied cleaning purge unwittingly just before bleeding. Some women like to create altars, or to change their altars for the time of bleeding. It can mean seeking out a place in nature that is special to you. Interpret this word in your own way. I think doing any of 'the allies' generates an internal sense of sanctuary or sacred space.

Sacred: Start to think of menstruation as sacred time, however that word speaks to you. Especially mark as sacred the point in the cycle that you most struggle with. Simply beginning to think this can have a quietly transformative effect. It is really a secret blessing of yourself, and I think as women you can't get enough of that.

Support: Get support during menstrual time and give superwoman a day off. Or as one woman suggested delegate, delegate, delegate. Can I say it any more clearly? Many menstrual tensions will bite the dust in the face of this one. And the positives of menstruation will naturally emerge.

Sleep: This is powerful spiritual practice and the most powerful of all for overworked women. It does wonders for your being at all levels and it seems women need more sleep coming into and when we bleed. Perhaps it's the extra dreaming we're after or simply that it is our natural time of rest and repair. Go for it.

HOLD THE CHARGE

It requires a discipline of awareness to hold feelings inside without suppressing, or necessarily acting on them but simply feeling their 'weight' and 'form', the way they snag, sting, heat, drive, stir, depress, exalt, sing, still. Of course we're going to speak out, cry out and crumble at times and a dose of all that is good too. However, learning to develop a curiosity for and capacity to hold the inner wildness that so wants to rock and disturb the apparent happy equilibrium of our lives allows both a real maturity of spirit to evolve and the possibility of the ineffable to touch us.

In that activity of awareness and containment without seeking speedy resolution, our being is worked on and activated, and the acreage of our souls expanded. It is as though more inner space is being carved out, and in that spaciousness the Great Mystery can make itself known in us. We also acquire greater psychological maturity. The more inner space we can sustain the more inner flexibility we have to deal with life's vicissitudes, to know what is for public expression and what to contain inside as our own private inner work. As a result we will be less reactive and more strategic and proactive in our expression. Increased inner spaciousness means greater freedom. It also creates a greater sense of aliveness and creativity and enhanced psychic and intuitive ability. This is your very own inbuilt wisdom growing process in action.

VALUE YOUR SELF

It can take courage to let go of your agendas, to step into the unknown and to surrender. Initially it can almost feel catastrophic, or at the very least a little strange and uncomfortable. It can also feel like you are going against the current of every one else. You probably are and that's the point. At menstruation you're stepping out of the normal, that is mainstream, consensus trajectory and all the usual expectations people have of you. It might feel like you are rocking the boat to stay close to the demands of this deep inner rhythm, but it is a necessity that you do. Tension isn't bad it's the *prima materia,* the basic ground, of the creative process. So far this sounds like quite a lonely project and I do think that accessing the power of menstruation requires being removed from the externalized, objectified world. However it does not have to be a lonely place. You may be separated from everyday life but you may find yourself entering a wonderful space of expansion, connection and possibility: a place blessed with love and belonging.

YOUR UNIQUE EXPERIENCE OF THE CYCLE

There is absolutely no right way to experience the cycle. What will unfold through this course are ideas to get you going on your own journey of discovery. Your experience will depend on:

Your individual temperament: you are all so singular and will inevitably bring a different emphasis or angle to this work. Let your singularity of character be the lodestone as you engage with this material.

Your overall health: the state of your immune system, digestion, energy levels and any chronic health problem are finely woven into this story. The poorer your immune system the more heightened your experience may be in some cases.

Life circumstances: whether you are in a relationship or not, your status (work, family, society in general), in other words how much power/authority you feel you have; physical environment – pollution, electromagnetic radiation (EMR).

Age: at different stages of our lives different themes or needs dominate. The distinctive pattern of the cycle may also take a little time to establish itself after menarche and then as we approach menopause it starts to break down.

Degree of self-awareness, self-esteem and willingness to court the life of your body.

THE PARADOX PRINCIPLE

This work is full of paradox. How is it that that which has been created must be uncreated for creativity to be ever renewing? How much is our capacity to say "yes" to others predicated on our capacity to say "no" to them (and simultaneously "yes" to ourselves)? How much is our capacity for productivity dependent on having apparently 'non-productive' time, that is, rest and reflection? We rely so much on what is visible, active and 'out there' and need also to trust the dormant, the invisible and the numinous aspects of life. The cycle embodies the continuous process of beginnings and endings, birth and death, the eternal return that keeps everything alive. It is critical to develop an ironic imagination;[1] a capacity for delight in the abiding intelligence of contradiction, an imagination that can hold the tension of opposites without the need for resolution. It is this capacity you will need most as you navigate the mysteries of the Deep Feminine encoded in your being.

[1] The term 'ironic imagination' came from the writings of Robert Sardello on the work of soul.

THE BIG BLEED AND THE SMALL BLEED

I am not referring here to how much blood you lose at menstruation but rather to the fact that some periods can feel highly charged and others periods more low key. Rather like the difference between big dreams – dreams that are highly, significant, archetypal and even full of portent – and more mundane ones, some menstruations can feel of cosmic proportions that come out of nowhere and others more ordinary. I can never really account for these as I cannot account for big dreams. It is like a Grace, though I do suspect that the more you consciously work with the cycle the more likely you are to have big bleeds. It is also worth paying attention to the phases of the moon, as this will also affect the intensity of your experience of menstruation.

> Now it's time to start on Month 1 of **The Woman's Quest**.
>
> Happy questing!

JOIN THE COMMUNITY OF QUESTERS

There is a **Woman's Quest community website** where you can share your experiences with other women from around the world. It's invitation only. If you'd like to join, email me at: *info@womensquest.org* and I will send you an invitation. Look forward to seeing you there!

Session 1:

Getting to know your cycle

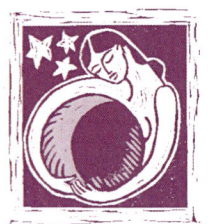

Our focus

This month you'll be getting to know your cycle, developing a curiosity for and establishing a quiet intimacy with it so that you can start to grasp the tendencies, strengths and opportunities of your menstrual month. For those of you who already feel you have a familiarity with your cycle, use this as an opportunity to come at it with fresh eyes, or simply deepen into it, sensing more texture and detail.

You'll be cultivating the skill of allowing – not much action but simply a deep allowing for the cycle to present itself to you. This will be the focus of the first two sessions.

Simply being in touch with the cycle has its own quiet magic and inner sweetener for our lives. At first it may be barely noticeable, but if you can sustain the process of attention you'll be building an inner sanctum, the breeding ground for that most seditious of forces, love. By this I mean a respect for yourself that casts its glow everywhere. This is the basic spiritual practice for your menstruating years: ever present, undemanding, except, of course, if you suffer from difficult menstrual problems. It will also inform and deepen all other self-development and spiritual practices you may wish to do.

Stillness

Hang out, potter (this can create a lovely inner stillness), lie down, do nothing, stare into space, just find someway to STOP mentally as well as physically.

What you need to do

STEP 1: LOOK AFTER YOURSELF

Regard the act of awareness and the charting of your cycle as self-care activity. This month also focus on the ally of *stillness*. Practice moments of stillness through the month but particularly when you are coming into and during menstruation.

In ensuing sessions I introduce dietary and other health suggestions but for this month simply enjoy the act of observation.

STEP 2: OBSERVE AND GATHER

As you go about your day-to-day business, keep an inner attention quietly present to the sense of the cycle. This is not necessarily an experience of the biological aspects of the cycle, although you may indeed feel such things as the ovary releasing its egg for that month or the proliferation of mucus around ovulation, which can feel special in itself. Rather, it's an imaginative and feeling sense. The attention you give is more a gentle sideways kind of look, a sensing rather than deliberate focusing. Just notice the general tone and mood of your inner state, feelings and sensations. Cultivate an inner stillness and imagine you can feel the rhythm and currents of your body. You don't have to be on the job every minute of the day, just check in now and then.

Naturally, you'll have ups and downs through the day that aren't connected to your menstrual cycle. Sometimes you may have particularly challenging life circumstances over and above the usual day-to-day life issues that will dominate everything and affect your experience of the cycle. Just keep observing and gathering and stay close to the deeper parts of your being whatever your situation.

At the end of each day record your observations in your **journal** and on your **Menstrual Dreaming chart**. Did you experience any of the following?

1. Particularly memorable dreams and times of dreaminess
2. Strong intuitive, psychic or synchronous moments
3. Heightened feeling, absence of feeling
4. Feeling of connection, lack of connection, desire for intimacy/aloneness
5. Feeling good about yourself/feeling yucky about yourself, comfortable in your own skin/not comfortable in your own skin
6. Sexual/not sexual
7. People's reactions to you/your reactions to people
8. 'Good' mother/'Bad' mother feelings
9. Feelings about your life, work, relationships
10. Ability/inability to act/initiate
11. Toughness/gentleness
12. Wants and needs – emotionally, spiritually, relationally, food cravings, sexual desire, ambitions
13. Physical changes.

Reflect on your observations at the end of 'the month'

1. What have you learnt about your cycle/yourself this month?
2. How do you feel *within* yourself having sustained this quiet inner attention for the month? What are you noticing about yourself and the world?
3. What part of the cycle do you feel most comfortable with?
4. What part of the cycle most unsettles or unseats you? How could you take care of yourself at that time? What would help you? Plan to give yourself a little of that next month. Write in your diary approximately when this phase will next occur with instructions on what to do or give yourself.

In your charting you might also want to include the four quarters of the moon. If you wish, you can also note physical changes including temperature (using the special basal ovulation thermometer) and mucus changes for contraception and conception purposes, although these observations are not essential to complete this course.
(For detailed information on how to do this and the appropriate charts, see *The Contraception Kit* by Francesca Naish and Jane Bennett. For more details go to: **www.nfmcontraception.com**).

17

Session 2:

Mapping the four phases of the cycle

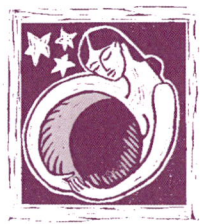

Our focus

In this session you'll be adding another layer of observation of your cycle as you tune in more acutely to the different phases of it and the intelligence at work in those phases. You'll also become aware of the transitions from one state to another.

There are two poles to a woman's cycle – ovulation and menstruation. Around each of these poles is a psychological and spiritual field of consciousness. It's like having two alternating currents of energy within your being which I call ovulatory mind and menstrual mind. Each pole offers different modes of intelligence and ways of being.

When you're in one mode, the other doesn't disappear. It is more a case of what is amplified, or brought to the fore.

As you move from one pole of the cycle to the other you go through a transitional phase where you're neither quite one nor the other. For most of us there is no clear demarcation line. It's rather like the day dawning, the light gradually getting stronger until midday or high noon and then shifting slowly, going down again into night. Night is menstrual consciousness and midday is ovulatory consciousness. There are the sacred moments of dawn – night crossing into day, and dusk – day crossing into night. These are the transitional, or liminal times, when we're in neither one nor the other. The dawning 'hours' of the menstrual cycle are pre-ovulation and the evening 'hours' (for some it can feel like far too many days!) are the premenstruum. These liminal or transitional times also have their own character, purpose and opportunities, so you might also think of them as distinct phases too. They are rather like the seasons of the year: pre-ovulation is the spring, ovulation the summer, premenstruum the autumn and menstruation the winter of the cycle.

Slowness

This means moving at the actual pace of your being and not everyone else's timing. You may feel considerably slowed down, but don't be fooled for one minute into thinking that you're somehow less capable or productive. Actually you're profoundly connected to yourself – now that's power.

What you need to do

STEP 1: LOOK AFTER YOURSELF

1. Add the ingredient of *slowness* to the premenstrual days, but particularly during the day or two before bleeding, and during day one and two of the period. Plan your schedule to allow for this.

2. Plan to give yourself at least 10 per cent (that is, a small dose) of one thing that would be symbolic of you caring for yourself better at 'that time of the month.'

STEP 2: MAPPING THE PHASES

As in the previous session, you'll be staying close to the deeper currents of atmosphere and feeling within you. While there are hormonal changes happening in the body that accompany or initiate your mood shifts, energy or impulse, it's not necessary to know precisely what the hormones are doing. Rather, you need to feel deeply your inner *sense* of things, and to chart that.

Pre-ovulation

As you emerge from the days of bleeding when the charge of the bleeding time has eased, notice your inner state, the quality of your connection to the world. Pay attention to your dreams, tastes, activities, level of activity and confidence. Deeply feel into these few days, the inner quality, even as your outer self may have to go about 'business as usual', with little regard for this level of subtlety.

- What is the word or image that describes this time?
- What is the quality of your energy like?
- How are you connecting/relating to the world?
- What is your tendency at this time particularly if you didn't have to think of others?
- What are the possibilities of this time?

Use your journal and the menstrual dreaming chart as you feel to record this.

Ovulation

When in the ovulatory phase you may not know the exact moment of ovulation itself, however for a number of days you will know yourself to be around that 'time' that is close to or soon after. Use the above questions again to flesh out this space.

Premenstruum

The cycle turns and tips into another space called the premenstruum. For some of you that world announces itself quite acutely for others it is a gradual creeping up. Again ask yourself the above questions.

Menstruation

For some this will announce itself with the arrival of bleeding. I also think it can announce itself anything from a few hours to a day or even two before the bleeding. There is an extraordinary moment of what I can only call 'suddenly feeling separated from the world,' detached, in another space. You may not identify it until after the fact. You may also tie that moment in with the premenstrual experiences. It really doesn't matter. The main task is fine-tuning your awareness. This fine-tuning is helping you to build the container to handle the charge of the elemental forces, to enter the depths of yourself. Again respond to the above questions.

STEP 3. EXPLORE FURTHER

Now, for each phase, consider the following questions and note your thoughts in your journal.

1. What's positive or good about each phase?
2. What do you find are apparent limitations, or not so useful aspects of each phase? What does this tell you about the kind of person you are?
3. What are you able to achieve/not achieve? What can/can't you do easily?
4. How are you relating to people?
5. Are you drawn to particular sorts of literature, music or other interests in the different phases? How might this speak to you?
6. What is/are the quality of your relationship/s like at these times.
7. What is your experience of yourself?
8. Who are you at ovulation/menstruation?
9. What kind of acknowledgement do you get from the world (the bigger society and your more immediate world) for this way for being? What does this tell you?
10. How do you know you're in the ovulatory/menstrual mind?
11. Are you more comfortable with yourself in the ovulatory world or the menstrual world? If so what do you think is the reason for that?

These questions are just to get you going. You can add your own or discard the ones that don't work for you. Feel free to follow your own riffs.

STEP 4. CHART YOUR MENSTRUAL DREAMING

Fill in the diagram on this page with key words for the different phases of the cycle. Try to get a sense of the distinctive character of the two poles (ovulation and menstruation) that create the dynamic tension for your evolution. For the artistically inspired among you, draw a larger diagram and use colour and imagery to fill it in.

You could also take 4 large sheets of paper or card and create a collage of images and words for each phase of the cycle. It's as though you are creating a map of your cycle like those colourful medieval ones that had comments like 'there be monsters.' (PS: for us it would read 'there be unlived or unembodied power').

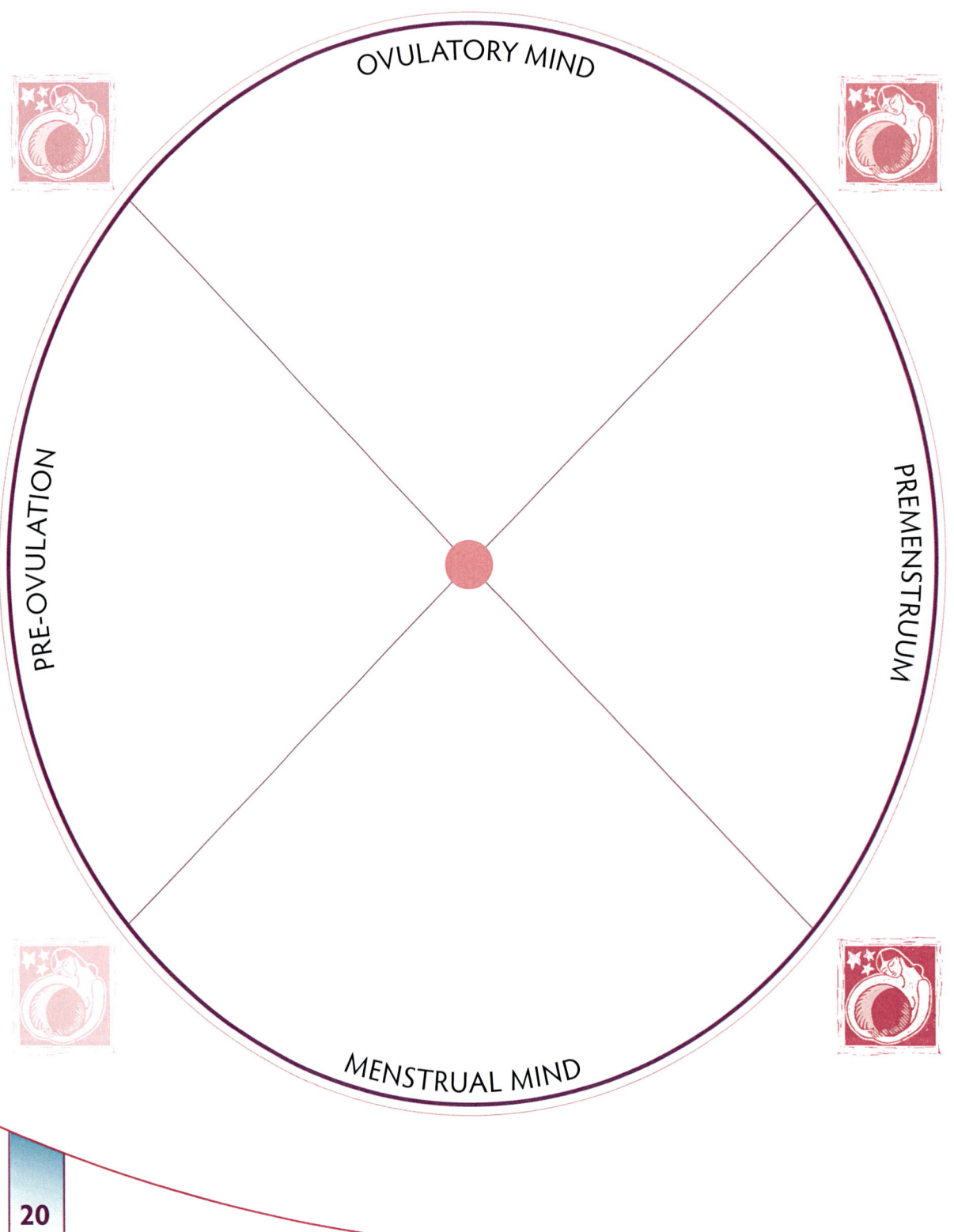

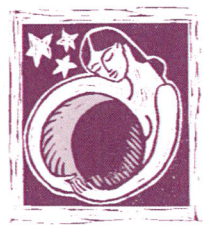

Session 3:

Inner work and the premenstruum

Our focus

The premenstrual phase is a time when we learn about and strengthen our capacity to handle our power. It is the time of heightened feeling and sensation, of greater complexity and depth, force and vulnerability, chaos and loss of control. The primordial forces are making their presence felt. It is the time when our deep self speaks more strongly, when the World itself comes knocking and asks something of us. And it is the time of disruption to the usual mode of operating, the interrupter of the status quo, with which comes the opportunity to re-evaluate, sort, face up to, edit, hone, complete, feel the deeper pulse, agitate and change things.

That which has been unattended to, sidelined, unspoken, or unacknowledged speaks premenstrually. It's almost inevitable that this will occur to some degree for it is the natural time for completions and cleaning up (literal and non-literal) and to agitate for change. However, if the experience is very intense or extreme, then you're getting clear signals that you may be avoiding or denying something in your overall life.

The premenstrum is the time when you're invited into a new knowing but, unless you're ready and able to ride the often powerful, critical and provocative consequences of speaking from this space, it may not always be the best time for you to deal with that new knowing. Heads can roll! Of course, sometimes we speak out even when we'd rather not say anything. And sometimes it's just the best time to deal with things because of that. Above all be curious. Take in all that's happening. If your reactions are extreme, remove yourself, write and reflect. I'm not recommending you lash out at people, it's not a licence to abuse others – I am asking you to accept that there is something immensely valuable happening.

Regard the premenstrum as sacred time regardless of whether it's good or bad for you. The more comfortable you are with it, the easier it will be to ride that great premenstrual liberator and trouble shooter and use it wisely. It's potent and, when not engaged with consciously, it becomes the time of serious distress, rather than the time of opportunity, self-awareness and evolution. Your task is to handle this elemental essence. It is real, meaningful and a critical part of the integrity of your being.

What you need to do

STEP 1: LOOK AFTER YOURSELF

1. Keep your quiet attention to the cycle going. By now this will feel more natural and easy.

2. Practice anointing the premenstrual transitional phase as *sacred* time. Interpret that loosely for yourself. Even just saying to yourself "I'm in my sacred time right now," will affect how you conduct business. I'd also still encourage you to hold on to the practice of *stillness* and *silence* as you bleed. They all go together well.

> ### Sacred
> *Start to think of menstruation as sacred time, however that word speaks to you. Especially mark as sacred the point in the cycle that you most struggle with. Simply beginning to think this can have a quietly transformative effect. It is really a secret blessing of yourself, and I think as women you can't get enough of that.*

STEP 2: ATTEND TO INNER WORK

You already know some things about this phase, so this month you'll use that knowledge while also mining for more as the premenstruum comes around again.

1. What happens in your premenstrual phase? What opens up in you and what are you opened to?

2. What do you like in yourself in this phase? What are your strengths here? Can you handle them effectively? If not, why not?

3. What are you tripped up by, what are your Achilles' heel moments or issues? How could this be a potential strength or opportunity for something else?

4. What is difficult or troubling?

5. What are you able to glean about your needs and deeper self, about what might be missing or not working in your life?

As you answer the questions at left, also ponder the following:

1. What must you address whether in yourself or in the world?

2. How might you approach the next month?

3. What do you need to honour in yourself?

4. How can you honour that spirit that disturbs?

STEP 3: MAKE NOTES TO YOURSELF

In your journal write down what you are going to do in the next cycle to empower yourself – just a few items and keep it simple. For example:

> **Note to self:**
>
> Catch myself doing something right
>
> Give up door mat status with husband/children/best friend/work colleague
>
> Set clearer boundaries with 'x'
>
> Tell 'y' what I want/assert my needs instead of giving in to their agenda
>
> Listen more
>
> Go to bed before 10 pm
>
> Reduce car use to help environment
>
> Write letter to my member of parliament regarding . . .
>
> Have breakfast at least 5 mornings a week
>
> Have a creativity 'date' with myself
>
> Make the 3 days before I bleed alcohol free
>
> Risk one thing different this month
>
> Buy a bunch of red roses for myself for menstruation
>
> Check in with my journal and this course before going to bed each night even if it's just to read the notes

(And so it goes – you get the idea)

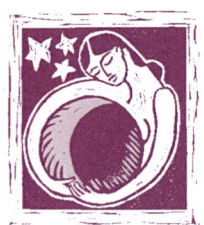

Session 4:
Losing it, using it – power and the premenstruum

Our focus

Along with the fall of your defences premenstrually, your polite socialised self bites the dust. An elemental energy is released. It's your life force, your own deep, wild instinctual, authoritative essence. It's like a genie coming out of the bottle – only this one is not so much granting you wishes, rather it's a force of revelation urging you act on or manifest that revelation yourself. The fog lifts and you can see through things; your tongue is loosened; you can't hold back your feelings or ideas; and intuition and instinctual knowing are heightened. For those of you for whom the fog doesn't lift, that, is you often feel foggy, or very internal and dreamy, your time will come in Session 11.

Irritability, anger, depression, pickiness, frustration, outspokenness, forcefulness, drive, woundedness, feeling overwhelmed, wildness and 'losing it' are some indications of power in all its guises rankling and wanting out. In fact, I dare to say that the emotional messiness of the premenstruum is all connected with power, including the feelings of woundedness and overwhelm. This may seem strange as the latter are associated with weakness yet hidden in that experience is an aspect of power that you don't yet know how to live out. It is a high sensitivity. (You will explore this more in Session 7.)

The rise of the menstrual elemental force begins to activate that which has been deadened, denied, ignored, or not lived out in you. It's also an ecstatic energy in the making. It's not unlike the feeling of having consumed just one too many drinks. You're not drunk, but an inhibition has fallen away and you're letting things rip a little. Learning how to feel, hold and ride this ecstatic force is the work of your menstruating years.

> ### Simplicity
> *Just do the basics of daily living now, no complicated cooking for family or organising some great project. Keep it simple.*

What you need to do

STEP 1: LOOK AFTER YOURSELF

Add a dose of *simplicity*, along with *stillness*, *slowness* and *sacredness*, when you bleed. Avoid alcohol ideally all month but particularly before and during bleeding.

STEP 2:
REFLECT ON YOUR POWER

How do your premenstrual experiences speak to you about power? What kinds of dreams are you having, are there repeating themes? And what do they tell you about your relationship to power?

STEP 3: GET TO KNOW THE GENIE

Feel the first initial agitations or awakenings of the 'wild genie,' the elemental force working you, right through to bleeding. For some there can be a strong sense of a 'loosening of the moorings' – a feeling of abandon or wildness somewhere in those days or hours before bleeding. Menstruation brings its own unique taste of this energy too. Even if you're in constricted circumstances, for example, bringing up a young child on your own or working in a very conservative or oppressive environment, where you need to constrain that feeling of wanting to 'abandon,' how does it make its presence known anyway?

This exercise is a deep process of sustained awareness and meditation. Notice what's happening and feel it at a deep visceral level. Relish it, even if it's a bit discomforting, and work on containing it to some extent. Containing doesn't mean not expressing your feelings, but it will help you to bring more discernment to what you say or do. You're living into this genie energy more thoroughly than previously when your focus was on the content of the cycle. Now you're concerned with the process underlying all the content. The act of awareness and sustained feeling of your experience carves out greater inner spaciousness and with that a stronger feeling of presence.

You can experience an ecstatic force at menstruation but if you don't have sufficient care for this feeling of abandon or wildness you can end up feeling out of control in a way that's not good. The work of awareness and containment builds the capacity to 'lose it' in an ecstatic sense rather than in a chaotic, distressing sense.

Note your observations in your journal.

STEP 4: ALLOW FOR SOME 'LOSING IT' TIME

And a little 'losing it' is also healthy! Although this might sound like I'm contradicting myself, some 'losing it' – allowing yourself to let go – is one reason why the cycle is good medicine physically and psychologically. So give yourself some 'losing it' time as well. This is a moment when you stop holding it all together and give up and walk away. It might be the need for a weep, to be a dag, let chaos reign, let your impatience show, get really stroppy, or break all your own rules. Enjoy.

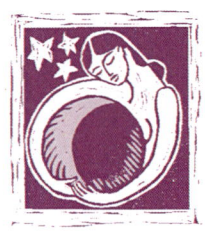

Session 5:
Power and the critic

Our focus

Somewhere in those days before bleeding there is *that* archetypal moment when our patience and tolerance levels drop precipitously low and out comes the inner critic. This can be directed at both others and ourselves. This critical energy is a challenging, sometimes difficult presence, but it's also an agent of change like no other. Learning to meet and deal with this inner figure is a training ground for greater self-acceptance and inner strength to handle this thing called power.

A vital part of getting stronger is learning to handle criticism, both that which you deliver to yourself and that which you receive from others. Learning to deal with the critic in all its manifestations is liberating. Not wishing to overstate the obvious, its role is to be critical so don't expect niceness. It's a power broker, even a potential leader in you wanting to come out, to help you grow. Ultimately the critic is presenting you with an opportunity to claim 'yourself' – to love and live the fullness of who you are. We will explore this further in the next session.

Softness

Practice genuine tenderness and generosity with yourself. No tough regimes. Although these might be good or necessary to have, in this moment they work against the exquisite subtlety and intimacy that is possible at menstruation.

Facing the critic each month is a 'calling to account' moment. You have to face yourself. The more you can do this the more confident you will become. The critic acts like a sword cutting through the crap. It helps you clean up your emotional as well as practical business each month. You may find yourself editing, pruning, cleaning up and refining both the inner and outer to some degree. This can be highly productive as well as a little humbling. The challenge is not to let it prune you too fiercely and leave you feeling crippled or for you to be pruning others too fiercely. This is neither productive nor good.

The stronger the critic the stronger the potential power in you, so take it as compliment if you have an excessively tough inner voice. Your critic has big plans for you and needs you to be strong so it sets you tough tasks that will demand a concomitant force in you to meet it. If you can meet it, over time you forge psychological muscle – discernment, clarity, focus, love and considerable energy. When you don't face it, it can be destructive of yourself and others.

What you need to do

STEP 1: LOOK AFTER YOURSELF

Since we are dealing with the critic this month practice the ally of *softness*, that is kindness and gentleness towards yourself in the premenstrual sacred time: for example give yourself the benefit of the doubt, drop some things off the 'to do' list, don't push yourself, treat yourself.

Go out of your way to acknowledge yourself in some way. If this is not easy ask a friend to tell you things she admires in you. Offer your friend the same admiration too. Build the positive credits in the bank account of your psyche. Affirm wastefully. Catch yourself doing something right.

Enjoy your food whatever it is. Catch the inner running commentary that says I should or shouldn't be eating this or that. And really make a choice to enjoy fully whatever you are eating. (Don't worry, next month you can go back to giving yourself a hard time for eating junk if you want to!) If you have a tendency to eat foods that you'd rather not in the premenstrual time, plan for it and give yourself some of what you crave without judgment. Give yourself the chocolate cake, chocolate or whatever it is. Give yourself the best. Do it in style, do it with awareness, revel in every delicious mouthful.

STEP 2: TIPS FOR HANDLING THE CRITIC

1. Value your cycle – this is a gesture of affirmation towards yourself, and is both strengthening and healing and an essential step in strengthening your capacity to face the critic.

2. Accept that you will encounter this figure monthly and that you need to face it. In other words, be prepared. Know your vulnerable times regarding criticism in general and avoid overexposure then. This is another act of self-kindness.

3. Start to pay more attention to how you speak to yourself at that time. What is this critical voice in you saying to you? This is a wake up call. Begin in small ways to face the issues. If you heed it you will get stronger and if you don't heed it the critic will get stronger.

4. The critic can bring home some painful home truths. One way to disarm it is to agree with it. This doesn't mean you agree with everything it says, but you may find at least one percent of truth in its words. Acknowledge that and you'll feel something shift. The way to feed this monster is to avoid or deny its accusations. Or equally to try and overly justify your position. Justification can be fuel to the fire of the critic.

5. Listen to those big existential questions the critic throws you just before bleeding. What's your life about? Are you on track? Are you doing what you really want to be doing? Are you facing things you should be? Is your relationship working? Or, why aren't you in a relationship? Face the questions as best you can. At times such critical probing can be debilitating, so it also helps to have allies such as reality checks from friends, and a loving and firm therapist or counsellor.

6. Seek support, ideally with a therapist who appreciates the psychology of the cycle, when you feel you're 'losing it' as there may be more complex forces at work than can be dealt with in this course. Sometimes the critic can be so intense we don't actually realise it's the critic at work. We may be feeling an incredible depression or despair, even suicidal, or extremely angry. In the premenstruum old traumas and chronic troubles can be re-activated and highlighted.

STEP 3: ENGAGE THE CRITIC

- What challenging issues come up for you premenstrually?
- What are you critical of in yourself and others?
- What do you give yourself a hard time about?
- What are you being asked to face in yourself?
- What is your inner critic asking of you?

Write freely about this – notes for your own consumption only.

Create a character called 'my inner critic'
If you could imagine your inner critic as an actual person what would it look and sound like and how does it conduct its 'business.' Draw an image of it and write about it. If you could imagine being more like this figure, how could this figure be helpful or useful in your life? (Yes, useful) And what are its limitations?

Have a conversation with your critic
Write out a conversation between you and your critic. Listen to what it has to say and respond back. Go for details as critics are weak on the fine print and love the grand sweeping condemning statement.

Take action
In the coming month address what you learn from facing the critic. Make some movement, however small, in the direction you wish to go, or situation you want to improve.

Sample conversations with the critic

Here are some sample conversations with the critic, but do remember that conversations with our inner critic aren't usually as tidy as the first two. The third is a real conversation from the journal of a woman called Lucy that spontaneously emerged as she was dealing with emerging feelings of dread. She was remembering events from the past and feeling a growing contempt towards herself. But as she kept writing something else emerged – a re-empowerment through naming the critic and taking it on.

SCENARIO 1

Critic: *Nothing's working in your life, you're a failure.*

You: What do you mean, nothing's working?

Critic: *Well, you're in a job that's going nowhere. You haven't got a relationship.*

You: It's true I'm not happy with my job and it's true that I'm not in a relationship but that doesn't make me a failure. I'm very good at my job, committed and hard working. I've got great friends and am a good friend. I've a lot to be grateful for. I do take your point that something isn't working for me right now but just because I haven't managed to get out yet doesn't mean I'm a failure it just means I've failed to find another job, so back off. And I am making a note to myself to really start looking for a new job.

SCENARIO 2

Critic: *God, you're an idiot, why aren't you like everybody else? Why do you have to be so reactive, what's wrong with you?*

You: Whoooah. That's quite a mouthful critic. Let's start with I'm an idiot. What have I done that was so stupid?

Critic: *Well, you mouthed off to 'x,' you got worked up and emotional.*

You: You mean I lost it a bit?

Critic: *Yes.*

You: Well I was speaking my mind and yes, I did get angry and would have preferred not to, but so be it. Getting angry doesn't mean I'm an idiot, it simply means I expressed my feelings very strongly. And to be honest it felt rather good.

Critic: *Yeah, well you looked like you were losing it and that's a stupid thing to do. You looked stupid.*

You: Sounds like you think losing it is somehow shameful. I'm not ashamed of getting angry. In fact, if anything, I'm unhappier with myself for having put up with that crap for so long.

Critic: *Well you really shouldn't have put up with it of course. You should have spoken out ages ago.*

You: It seems I can't get it right with you. Firstly you're bailing me out for speaking out and now you're nailing me for not having done it sooner. There's no pleasing you that's for sure. So back off. I'm doing the best I can. I'm human.

Critic: *Yeah, well you could end up with no friends at all if you don't get it right.*

You: Yes, critic, part of the risk of being alive is that I could put my foot in it. I suspect the world won't come to an end and all my friends won't abandon me but let's just see. I expect I'll survive, maybe I could make new and better friends. Things are never quite as bad as I imagine they're going to be. I need to remind myself of that.

Critic: *Harrumph.*

And that real conversation

" ...There is absolutely no point whatsoever in going over these things (of the past) – none at all... Can't think of any point whatsoever it's just foolish behaviour – get that critic? O contemptuous one, it's foolish behaviour, it's worse it's a waste of time, it's boring, it's all the same old things from the past, there's nothing interesting or engaging or enlightening in any of it, so you might as well go away and find something useful to do because this is not it. There is nothing at all useful in this bullshit, boring time wasting behaviour. It's distracting. The worst thing is it's distracting from the present. It ought to be a criminal offence; you ought to be locked up. So stop it. And given that we are one we'd better work on this relationship seeing as how you can't get locked up separately from me. So what are we are going to do? Respect. We have to get some mutual respect going, we have to get some mutually aligned objectives, we have to get some trust and not be undermining each other. OK. So that's 3 things: 1. Respect, 2. Aligned objectives, 3. Trust and not undermining. OK let's work on 2. Objectives must be to help me to be the best person I can be – that involves encouragement, praise, giving direction, *constructive* criticism and not dredging up the past as a punishment. Constructive is to assess something I've done, see what could be done better – do the steps. *(Here she is referring to the 12 steps of AA).* Steps around defects of character and making amends and ultimately handing the whole lot over to god, to the great creator – to reweave them into new patterns. Yes, I get it, that's the constructive thing you can do, bring these things to light. Defects or bad behaviours or in fact usually mistakes, and hand them over to god to be dealt with, so it's a purging, not hanging on to the negative things and blowing them out of all proportion – good. That's really excellent. Then Respect will come from our cooperation in working towards our objectives and seeing our parts in that and Trust also will come from doing it and getting results. Not undermining is a decision we must make, an agreement that we will not undermine each other. OK. "

Session 6:

The bitch – your inner power broker

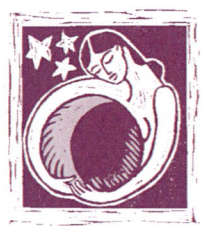

Our focus

Some of you might think of this 'bitch' energy as 'losing it' – enter the tough talking, assertive, provocative, knowing, sometimes angry figure that so many of us encounter premenstrually and often end up apologising for later. Otherwise known as the bitch or Babe In Total Control of Herself, she is a potent combination of that elemental force and the critical energy, she is a power broker in the making and not to be apologized for.

She has a wonderful instinctual, embodied intelligence that can sense bullshit a mile off and doesn't pull her punches. There's a fearless, sassy, 'look at me in the wrong way and I'll eat you alive,' sexually provocative edge to her that's really potent. And she'll get you into trouble if you don't understand and value her presence. As you learn to harness her force you'll feel a powerful detachment that allows you to be a penetrating truth speaker and change agent or activist. In that detachment you can become more truly a voice for something much bigger than yourself, for the World.

In some women she is incredibly pronounced and in others more muted. You may not experience her in quite the totality that I'm describing here but you may see aspects of yourself, equally there may be features that I haven't captured – let your inner sense of this figure teach you.

While I feel it's very important not to apologise for this figure, power is a double-edged sword and, yes, you might be abusive and hurtful and indeed may want to apologise for that. She is *not* a license to abuse. But, don't dismiss it as 'just premenstrual' because that also dismisses the content of what you say and diminishes your intelligence. People don't have to know you are in your premenstrual phase – that belongs in your 'notes to self' list to be more aware of this energy and learn to handle it better.

What you need to do

STEP 1: LOOK AFTER YOURSELF

Go slow on the alcohol again this month – alcohol and the bitch are a volatile combination. And avoid sugar. This doesn't mean you can't have sweet foods but it needs to be naturally sweet or sweetened (i.e. with fruits, dried fruits, rice malt, maple syrup). You can reduce your need for 'sweets' by eating a mineral rich, nutritionally dense diet that includes lots of vegetables (especially green leafy ones), some fruit, animal fats from organic or pasture fed sources (e.g. raw milk, yoghurt), and essential fatty acids from *fresh* raw nuts and seeds, cold pressed olive oil and fish oils.

Keep the allies of *stillness*, *sacred*, *simplicity*, *slowness*, and *softness* as features and add *sanctuary* this month. Interpret that in your own way. Slowing down, having some stillness and silence will automatically aid you in sanctuary. Think about what the word 'sanctuary' evokes for you and give yourself a dose of that.

Sanctuary

Create a feeling of specialness or sanctuary by having a sense of order in your physical environment, even if it's just your bedroom. Often women do have a frenzied cleaning purge unwittingly just before bleeding. Some women like to create altars, or to change their altars for the time of bleeding. It can mean seeking out a place in nature that is special to you. Interpret this word in your own way. I think doing any of 'the allies' generates an internal sense of sanctuary or sacred space.

STEP 2: GET TO KNOW YOUR INNER POWER BROKER

This month focus on this outspoken, provocative energy in whatever form it manifests for you *all month* long but particularly track it close to menstruation. Rather than seeing this as personal inner work, shift the angle and look on this energy as a real change agent, a leader. This is not dissimilar to what you did in Session 4 and 5 but with a shift in focus. In Session 5 the emphasis was more on facing yourself. Now you are concerned with acting on that inner awareness, doing something about it. It's about acting for the world – your family, local community or the bigger world.

1. How is this power broker figure calling you to speak out?
2. What issues disturb or trouble you?
3. What are the potential ways you sabotage or censor this figure?

STEP 3: SPEAK OUT

Find a way this month to honour this provocative outspoken figure through some action or activity while also caring for the parts in you that are nervous about all this outspokenness. Actually, some of you may already be using this force but don't value what you do. You may even be criticising it as 'too much'. Drop the criticism and start relishing your outspokenness.

Make notes on your action and the outcome.

Session 7:
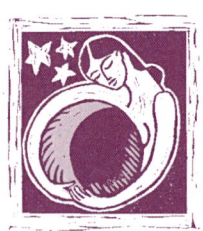
Power and vulnerability

Our focus

To be vulnerable is to be human. Being vulnerable means you are more open, with a heightened sense that allows you to feel more deeply and be moved. You are sensitive to and can be touched by life. Vulnerability allows you to enter a more expanded state of consciousness, connecting you to something beyond yourself. It allows you to experience love and greater subtly, beauty and depth of meaning. Vulnerability is intrinsic to emotional and spiritual strength. It opens you to the ecstatic, spiritual forces. Someone who is unable to feel vulnerable is emotionally dead. That emotional deadness shuts down your deeper intuitive and instinctual knowledge. While intellectually you may be able to function, you will be unable to truly engage with yourself and have deeply satisfying relationships. Without it you will become disconnected: a disconnection that can be the breeding ground for indifference and even violence.

Vulnerability is not something we associate with power. On the contrary it can feel pretty powerless to be vulnerable. You can feel overexposed, overwhelmed, chaotic, not in control, embarrassed, easily hurt and stupid – neither good nor powerful. However, as you let yourself feel unflinchingly into the spaces and issues that emerge through being vulnerable, and allow yourself be informed by them, you build the kinds of strength I described in the first paragraph.

The heightened state of awareness premenstrually, and at menstruation, that sometimes results in intense feelings of vulnerability is not a sign of weakness. Rather it is our unique monthly doorway through which we can step to strengthen our psychological and spiritual muscles. The simple act of valuing and caring for this heightened state allows access to the positives rather than leaving you feeling battered or overexposed by it.

While it's critical to have good boundaries – essential for a good sense of self – when those boundaries become too impregnable, you can become impermeable to influences from the world and to being 'touched.' Too strong a boundary builds egotism and separateness. Some permeability or vulnerability is vital to connect us to others. It also allows us to feel for the world and to feel the spiritual depths speaking to us. The premenstrual disturbance is not all personal – you may be feeling the mood of those around you or something connected to the condition of the world. You are like a lightning conductor picking up the unexpressed charge within your family, workplace or wider community. For example some women feel quite overwhelmed sometimes and cry very easily. I think they can feel the despair that exists in the world in many quarters – the hopelessness of some people's lives, wracked as they are by endless violence and loss of human rights.

I think of the premenstruum as a reawakening or revivifying of your senses and soul to the fuller reality of yourself and the world, a restoration of your full humanity. Sometimes that reawakening can feel like the painkiller wearing off after you've been to the dentist to have some dental work: tender, a bit sore but at least alive.

What you need to do

1. LOOK AFTER YOURSELF

Be thoughtful about diet. Avoid alcohol, particularly in the days leading up to your period, and reduce or eliminate coffee and sugar. These substances can really skew this high sensitivity and leave you feeling chaotic, weird or disconnected from yourself.

Drink plenty of purified water to stay hydrated. Continue practicing *softness* – kindness, kindness and more kindness with yourself as well as the other allies we have already drawn on. And add a dose of *solitude*. This also means some time without phones, computers, radio, TV or even music.

> **Solitude**
>
> *Make sure you get genuine empty space for yourself where you're not in relating mode.*

2. FOCUS INTO THE TENDER MOMENTS

Your task now is to meet and feel those vulnerable feelings and let them inform you. Curiously the act of meeting without doing anything can really shift things. That simple act creates greater soulfulness and inner strength that is priceless.

Mark clearly on your calendar or in your diary the most vulnerable times of your cycle and, as much as you are able, do less at that time. As it draws close, pace yourself, by moving at the pace of your body rather than your head. Stay close to that vulnerability, reduce stimulation, absolutely affirm the things that support you and say "no" to the things that don't. Don't push, bully or over expose yourself so that you can enjoy the positives of that vulnerability and not feel overwhelmed or bad about yourself. Absolutely make that time as sacred as you can.

- What did you experience or discover about yourself? What did it open you to?
- How are you feeling in yourself now that you have really allowed yourself to acknowledge and embrace that sensitivity? How are you feeling in your body?
- If you are in a relationship, what did you notice about the quality of your connection?

Session 8:

Liminality and creativity

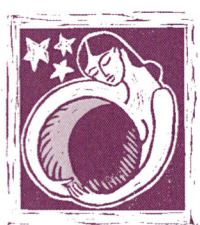

Our focus

Liminal space is transitional time and space where we're neither one thing nor the other. It is the gap between 'worlds,' between one state and another and between the mundane and the spiritual. We're in the process of letting go of one world, before the new has yet revealed itself. It's a 'changing of gears' time, both a dying and an emerging. We may feel more permeable or vulnerable. Feeling transitional for some can be overwhelming – a feeling of being out of control, lost, anxious, empty or depressed or at the very least 'not one's usual self.' And yes, you aren't your usual self, and that's the whole point – you're changing. It can also be a highly charged even ecstatic time.

There are the big liminal times such as puberty, pregnancy and birth, and menopause. Any major life transition, such as the beginning and ending of relationships, change of career, midlife transition (which for women is usually connected with menopause), and the death of a loved one are liminal moments that all hold great potency. Each change of season also brings such a moment and there are minor liminal moments in the day. The classic one is waking up, or making the transition from home to work or, equally, from work to home. You may notice that you have rituals for those thresholds such as feeling a need for a cup of coffee before you can settle into anything at the beginning of the workday, or even that drink as soon as you get home. Illness also puts us into liminal territory. Someone who is dealing with chronic health problems can feel chronically liminal, or marginal, in a way that can feel deeply isolating and meaningless.

Liminality is a deeply embodied experience for women because of the menstrual cycle as we move out of menstrual consciousness into ovulatory consciousness – the pre-ovulatory phase – and from ovulatory consciousness back to menstrual consciousness – the premenstruum. The premenstruum presents the greater challenge because it is the less attractive phase of the cycle – the dying or ending, when we may also want to pull away from others and be more internal, and for which we may usually get little support. Menstruation, while a place of arrival, is also liminal. We are neither pregnant nor fertile – no longer 'occupied' by others if you like. At such a moment we embody a role that is classically outside the accepted image of women, belonging to no one but ourselves. And a woman who is completely her own person is nothing but trouble!

Think of liminality as a portal through which you may travel to touch the timeless. Cultivating an awareness of it fosters creativity, a capacity to 'see through' things, to feel into the world behind worlds, and experience the deeper pulse that is 'working' us all. Spiritual practice is about cultivating that awareness beyond the mundane. Women are given the possibility of access to that 'world behind worlds' monthly through the dynamic of the cycle. The post-menopausal woman who has really lived and loved her cycle can stand firmly in the two worlds – the mundane and the sacred.

Think of liminal territory as a:

- Sacred time and space
- Window of opportunity
- Way of liberating your thinking
- Place to pause, reflect and collect yourself
- Time for dreaming and for creative ideas to flood in
- Opportunity to garner soul food and guidance for your life
- Time for magic, for scripts to be rewritten, the future restructured
- Place of power.

What you need to do

STEP 1: LOOK AFTER YOURSELF

Imagine the part that you most struggle with in the cycle as your power spot. For example, if you tend to get a headache on a certain day, feel a particular intense feeling, or get period pain, circle that day or days as your sacred time and give space to the thing that disturbs you. Imagine that holds teaching on your power in some way. Listen and observe. Write down any observations.

> **Silence**
>
> *Take some time without TV (especially have a news fast), music, computers, mobiles etc. Go into a cone of silence and let the zone of menstruation claim you.*

Add times of *silence* this month, particularly around menstruation. This is not dissimilar to *solitude*, although it's very interesting to enjoy silence when in the company of someone.

STEP 2: EXPLORING LIMINALITY FOR GREATER CREATIVITY

A. Your window of opportunity

The aim is not to be directed and focused, but to be in neutral gear, more allowing and fluid, while keeping a subtle quiet attention. It might appear as though nothing is happening. Nothing is good. And nothing isn't really nothing either. Something is happening but it's below your conscious awareness. It's simply good medicine to hang out now and then, and it can open a space for creative inspirations to come in.

When your concentration starts to wander after an extended period of focus, that's often a good signal that you may need to down tools for a few minutes and create a liminal moment. It's a window of opportunity for refreshing yourself.

When you're stuck with something at work, don't know the answer or what to do next, go walkabout around the office, daydream, go to the toilet, make a drink, stare out the window for a few minutes. This keeps your creative spirit alive. Don't even think about the issue. After a few minutes or so return to the matter in hand. You might surprise yourself with what emerges. Liminality has its own magic.

B. Experiment with liminal moments – hang out in them, court them, give yourself over to them.

- Take some still time at dawn or dusk. If you have the chance, literally watch as it changes from night to day and vice versa.

- Hang out in that half sleep/half wake moment of waking in the morning.

- Cooperate with the ups and downs of your energy through the day – when the downs come slow down, stop, 'check out' briefly even if it's only a matter of minutes. Don't force anything. The 'downs' can be windows of opportunity trying to happen.

- Factor in transitional time between activities in your day so you don't have to switch from one place, person or activity to another instantly.

- Consider too where you are in your life right now – it could be a transitional time overall because you're stepping into or out of a relationship, changing jobs, just completing a big project, going through menopause, experiencing your daughter entering puberty and having her first period.

- Focus on the liminal times of the menstrual cycle – consider what is the most intense, special or challenging moment for you and give yourself over utterly to it without any interruptions, tasks, distractions or contact with others. Surrender to its depths. You may really have to plan for this one. Do the best you can. Whatever you do will have an effect.

- Make notes on what you discover. What happens, or what is revealed, when you do the above? If you drive yourself hard and find it hard to stop, notice what stops you from going into those dreaming places.

- Menstruation is a particularly powerful liminal moment for inspirations and ideas to flood in – highly creative – but you do need to stop and hang out for awhile for that door of inspiration to really open.

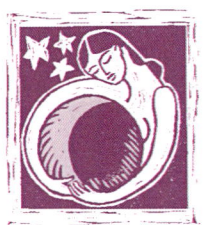

Session 9:

Intuition, guidance and meaning making

Our focus

Menstruation is a time of heightened intuition, which, over time, can mature into a high intuition increasingly available to you – a sustained intuitive mode of being. This is certainly the case during and after menopause. The more you attune to the cycle and let it educate you, the more this natural intuitive acuity will strengthen and the more able you will be to trust and act on it.

Intuition is that form of knowing that comes to you completely bypassing the normal rational pathways. You know without knowing why you know. Your whole being senses a rightness about the knowing. But your apparent intuitive flashes are not all foolproof; you need to also know the difference between intuition and wishful thinking and projection.

Intuition comes from a state of being – being present, caring for the rhythm of things both great and small and having an inner silence or stillness. The process of attuning to the cycle enhances intuition. To attune to our cycle we need to learn to ride and value our internal changing currents of mood and energy through the menstrual month; to experience the natural clearing out and surrender at menstruation that expands inner spaciousness, creating an inner stillness and silence. Repression of menstrual capacity works against your intuitive faculty sometimes turning up as distressing premenstrual symptoms.

The menstrual cycle is an inner referencing and guidance system. Through the movement of the cycle you experience different states of being that expose more of your inner world and overall wellbeing thus giving feedback on how you are travelling in life. Being in touch with this inner movement of the cycle enhances your senses and emotional intelligence. The movement draws you deeper into relationship with yourself. This activity is ultimately an act of love and works your faculty for intuition as well as your capacity for receiving guidance. It becomes a process of making meaning.

When consciously picked up and valued, menstruation's heightened state of consciousness becomes a marvellous opening to depth of feeling, imagination and spirit that will play out according to your own nature and calling in life. Heightened intuition and psychic ability allow you to tap deeper resources for guidance and wisdom in your lives.

Purpose and meaning are not commodities that can be just picked up off the supermarket shelf of life unfortunately. They come by more mysterious routes. It's almost as if you must create a space for them to be known. The premenstrual phase is a great undoing and unravelling. The process of being emptied out allows for the presence of grace to be known, for your life to feel pregnant with possibility and meaning, for you to become clearer about who you are and therefore what your calling or purpose may be. Menstruation, a time when you're delivered up to something greater, is a moment of deep alignment that can bring with it an enormous sense of meaningfulness. The more you attend to your overall experience of the cycle and the state of menstruation, the more you'll taste this. It's a kind of grace that can seep quietly into your whole life. Each of you may know this place in slightly different ways, but the underlying theme of meaning will gradually be undeniable.

What you need to do

STEP 1: LOOK AFTER YOURSELF

Focus on nourishing yourself psychologically and physically for the whole month and not just before your period. Make sure your diet is especially nourishing: include lots of green leafy vegies (make juices with them and add a carrot to make it more palatable); live food such as sprouts and fermented foods such as sauerkraut and yoghurt (without sugar and additives and, ideally, organic); nettle tea (a powerful mineral rich brew and a great friend to women), essential fatty acids in nuts and seeds such as linseed, sunflower seed and walnuts.

Enjoy the ally of *sleep* this month – get plenty of it. And particularly aim for a regular sleeping pattern, especially if you are a bit erratic about this. You don't have to stick to it after this month but for this month, really make an effort to establish a rhythm, just as an exercise. You might find you like it. For those of you who are mothers with babies or young children with broken sleep this will prove more challenging. But focus on it anyway. It might mean napping a bit when your children nap through the day rather that using that time to catch up on all the jobs. It may not be about getting more sleeping hours but simply more moments of rest or chilling out. Be creative as you surely already are as a mother.

> ### Sleep
> *This is powerful spiritual practice and the most powerful of all for overworked women. It does wonders for your being at all levels and it seems women need more sleep coming into and when we bleed. Perhaps it's the extra dreaming we're after or simply that it is our natural time of rest and repair. Go for it.*

STEP 2: FIND MEANING AND DIRECTION

Focus this month on your sense of meaning and purpose, or lack of it. Notice those times when you do feel a sense of purpose and then when it falls away. What nourishes meaning and what erodes it for you? Notice those times when you feel most alive and 'in the flow'. What do those moments reveal to you of your calling and direction in life?

As you come to the premenstrual phase, actively let go of who or what you think you are. You will know the moment when this is pertinent – it's when you start to feel slightly less than brilliant about yourself. Yes, that critic attack moment when self-doubts creep in and you feel overly critical, depressed, anxious or angry. At such a moment try just giving in. Giving in does not mean giving in to destructive practices towards yourself or others. It means simply feeling the despair, emptiness, pointlessness or whatever your particular undoing energy is and see where you end up. This can be especially helpful when you feel the first harbingers of the period announcing itself.

> Menstruation is the waking up moment from the numbing forces of consensus reality to rediscover your own truths. Pay attention to how you're being spoken to. Take dictation from the Divine. Take some time to record in your journal your responses to the following questions:
>
> - What arises in you through the transition and into the bleed?
>
> - What do you feel called to?
>   Don't judge what comes up just write freely. Hold the ideas inside you in the coming weeks letting them speak, take shape and fill out more (particularly in liminal moments notice what comes to you.)

STEP 3: PRACTISE THE 'BLEED ON IT' METHOD

If you have an issue you want to resolve, rather than 'sleeping on it' try 'bleeding on it'. Your menstrual cycle is a container of time to incubate an issue, and menstruation itself opens you to guidance from your deep being. Again, it doesn't involve trying to think about a solution, rather allowing the space for it to reveal itself. You can also take a number of cycles to deepen into a big life change – each cycle giving you another level of meaning and clarity.

Use the 'bleed on it' method for:

- Gaining more clarity on an issue.
- Looking for direction and meaning in general.
- Finding answers to specific questions and life issues.

The stages:

1. Set the intention.
2. Observe, gather and incubate.
3. Slow down, let go, empty out (at menstruation) and stay open to receive.

1. SET THE INTENTION

State clearly out loud, like a declaration to the universe, the problem or issue for which you seek guidance. This statement can be as simple or as grand as you want it to be. If you have the luxury of time, it's good to do this at the beginning of the cycle so that you have the whole month to let the issue incubate – especially important if you're dealing with big life challenges. You might also want to create a special ritual for the declaration, such as lighting a candle and meditating first.

2. OBSERVE, GATHER AND INCUBATE

Once you've made your declaration, let go of trying to solve the issue. As you go about your day-to-day business, simply pay attention, at a subtle level, to signs, signals and clues both from within yourself (including your feelings and dreams) as well as feedback from the World. Imagine the World is speaking to you on this issue.

You don't need to be overly focussed – on the contrary, a little forgetting is good. The attention you do give is more a gentle sideways look, a sensing as much as an actual seeing. Simply hold your observations inside you. If you find yourself getting anxious about still not having an answer (you might be someone who finds it difficult to take a back seat) remind yourself there's still time. If you harry yourself you'll be interrupting the very process that may give you the clarity you seek.

3. SLOW DOWN, LET GO, EMPTY OUT (AT MENSTRUATION) AND STAY OPEN TO RECEIVE

As you come into menstruation, slow down, do less, and let go to your natural tendencies instead of bullying yourself to keep going with what you'd normally expect of yourself. Move in a way that accommodates the changing rhythm and need of your body. Particularly as you bleed, give yourself some space to do nothing, to simply rest. Throughout this phase, stay open to what wants to be known in you. It can feel like an in-rushing of energy, an inspiration or a deep quiet certainty or knowing.

Day 3 or 4 of the cycle can be particularly illuminating, almost like a clear command to oneself. But to catch this moment of clarity you need to keep a degree of closeness to yourself, rather than getting lost in the 'busyness' of day-to-day life. Of course you can't drop all your tasks and responsibilities, but it's vitally important to claim space for yourself at this time, however meagre.

Premenstrually a 'no bullshit' voice can often come through with very clear instructions. You might want to act on it; however, harnessing that forceful spirit until you have bled may also mature the idea.

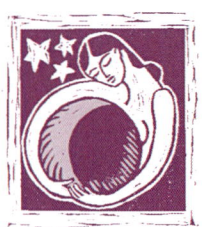

Session 10:

Intimacy and relationship

Our focus

The work of the cycle is ultimately the work of relationship: a coming into relationship with oneself and with the World. It's the work of coming into deep intimacy with Life in all her majesty. Menstruation is a portal to the Great Unknown or Mystery, the imminent presence of the Feminine. The experience of menstruation enfolds us and our sense of separation dissolves. It is an extraordinary blessing.

We have arrived at the heart of what I feel is the true power of menstruation – a capacity to taste an extraordinary intimacy. It's to feel the sweet caress of the most exquisite brush our metaphorical and literal skin, to relish its magnificence, to breathe it in and to be touched by it. The intimacy I speak of is an utter presence to the moment, to the particular. It's as though your defences have all fallen away and in that moment you Know and are Known. You have entered an inner sanctum, the Holy of Holies where the small self has fallen away and you experience a profound connection to All That Is. It is a moment of love and bliss. And if you are in a relationship, it can be a glorious opportunity to enter a more deeply loving place of union with your partner.

It was only in my forties that I began to notice this place of deep intimacy so acutely. It didn't occur every month with the same intensity. Some months were quite extraordinary, others more ordinary, but even then there was still something distinctly characteristic that occurred in the hours just before bleeding. Before my forties, as far as I can remember, I'd start to get restless, unable to concentrate and would want to get away from people in the twelve to twenty-four hours before bleeding. But then, when on my own, I would often feel a bit empty and lost. Later, I discovered this time held something else. It was as if I was being stolen away from normal life to enter a deep abiding silence, a feeling of awe that would have me almost gasping. I'd feel sweetly tender and full of love and bliss. It felt revelatory. It was also quite separate from the ecstatic feelings that occurred once the blood was flowing.

The poet, David Whyte, speaks of poetry as stealing one for revelation. And I realised that is precisely what happens at menstruation, we are stolen for revelation. The whole thrust of the premenstrual process is about removing us from the mundane world and tenderising us to receive revelation at menstruation, when the doors of perception are flung open.

This tender blissful phase just before bleeding struck me as enormously subtle and delicate. I could neither force nor program its presence, but simply court it. If the conditions were right it would appear, if not I might miss it. And I wasn't entirely sure what the conditions were. I began to tell women about it for I did not believe for one minute that this was unique to me. I just knew, and know, that it's a potential capacity in all menstruating women at bleeding time *if* a woman is interested.

So what are the conditions for this experience to occur? Unfortunately I can't give you the ten-step, foolproof guide. To do so would be to kill the very thing you're after. But I believe the practice unfolding through this course is your best means to know this place.

Generally speaking, avoid 'breakthrough' techniques, tough disciplines and even such things as sweat lodges at this time – while they may work for men, they deaden the faculty women need to enter this inner sanctum. This work of intimacy demands an exquisite subtlety of feeling, a deep exposure or nakedness to oneself and to the Other. It is an act of enormous self-acceptance. Generally speaking, we shy away from this intimacy even as we most yearn for it, because this 'nakedness' is most challenging.

This intimacy is not a private inner affair but becomes about a deep connection to All That Is. For me it's the secret ingredient in developing participatory consciousness – a consciousness that recognises we're all deeply interconnected and interdependent. And if you're in a relationship, and your partner is sensitive to the mysteries of the cycle, together it is possible to experience a deep tender union in those sacred hours leading into menstruation.

Your shifts of mood and energy through the cycle will also include a changing sexual desire that can enrich your union. Generally speaking you'll probably notice there are two moments when sexual charge is particularly high in the cycle: around ovulation – that's nature at work making sure we keep the species going – and at menstruation. Some women can feel an extraordinarily wild and provocative sexual force in the menstrual phase that is absolutely about unashamed sexual pleasure. Simply be curious about the intimacies of your own sexual charge through the month and relish them, whether you're in a relationship or not.

What you need to do

STEP 1: LOOK AFTER YOURSELF

Go without coffee, sugar or whatever your drug of choice is this month. I realise this may be easier said than done, so do your version of this. You might indeed be able to go without them, or it might mean reducing your intake or simply not imbibing them as you come into and during the bleed. The sugar craving can be singularly strong premenstrually. But, if you have been improving your diet steadily that craving, most likely, will have decreased.

Work on the theme of *sanctuary* again this month. It might mean creating a special environment to be in, or simply experiencing an inner sense of sanctuary. Give yourself permission to utterly *surrender* to who you want to be at menstruation as best you can within the circumstances of your life. Put aside any 'oughts' or 'shoulds' about what you think you're supposed to do or be, including any expectations you might have from doing this course. Privilege the state of menstruation above all other things this month.

> **Surrender**
>
> *Drop your endless agendas, aspirations and ambitions and momentarily 'die' (check out 'stillness').*

STEP 2: BUILD GREATER SELF-ACCEPTANCE

For intimacy and relationship to mature we need self-acceptance above all else. How can you be more loving and accepting of yourself this month? What gesture of affirmation can you make towards yourself? Where are you tough on yourself, unforgiving or overly critical? Make it a sacred charge this month to let go of one of those things that you give yourself a hard time about. Forgive yourself. Actively catch those constant niggly put-down thoughts and simply drop them. One way to do this is to say something positive in their place.

For example, if I'm about to say: "You idiot," or "That was dumb," I'll playfully say something to myself like "You're fine, you're great, you're doing okay." Even if you don't believe it, do it anyway; have some fun with it. Our internal level of put-down can sometimes be farcical, if someone spoke to us the way we speak to ourselves we'd be horrified. And if it were in the workplace they'd be had up for bullying. Choose a gesture of affirmation that's not too challenging, and then just do it.

STEP 3: CREATE SPACE FOR REVELATION

Mark in your diary when menstruation is due or roughly due. Minimise commitments at that time. As you get close to menstruation keep an inner awareness to that moment when you feel the blood is almost due. You will know that moment. Drop your agendas and do only what has to be done.

Move profoundly at the pace of your body/being and not your head. Ideally take some time to simply sit and do nothing. Being still and not engaging with others are the important keys to entering this zone of bliss on the cusp of bleeding.

STEP 4: CREATE SANCTUARY FOR RELATIONSHIP

Relationship needs sanctuary. If you're in a relationship, consider how can you strengthen a sense of sanctuary for the relationship itself.

Meditate on that word for you, discuss it with your partner; let something original emerge from your own reflections that you can actively do to nourish this sense of sanctuary. It's important that your partner has some appreciation of the nature of cyclical life and is comfortable with his or her own rhythms to some degree. The important ingredients here are tenderness and clarity about your own boundaries – what you're up for and not up for. You're drawing now on all that you have done to date through these sessions.

Tell your partner what you would like during menstruation and how they might help you to get the most out of this time. Use the menstrual time as a way of really connecting deeply with him or her. This is a delicate dance and, once again, I must emphasise the importance of slowness, not having heaps of things to do. You need space and time to *be* with each other – that is all.

STEP 5: REFLECT ON RELATIONSHIP

The changing nature of cycles opens you to different experiences of yourself and different ways of knowing. You are exercised in the art of change and with that the re-negotiation of who you are and your relationship to others. This constant movement becomes a wonderful instruction in the dance of relationship. Are you more aware now of that dance – the times when you feel very 'out there' in the world; the times when you want to withdraw to another kind of relationship, one with yourself; the process itself of moving from the outer to the inner relationship? Are you able to follow that movement towards and away from people or do you judge yourself as anti-social or selfish for wanting to be alone. That judgement doesn't support your unfolding wisdom. It erodes it. Read back through the notes you've been making throughout this course. Consider the following questions through the month:

- What have you learnt about relationship and the cycle through your study so far?
- What do you notice about the quality of your connections with others through the month?
- What does the cycle teach you about your relationship with yourself and with others?
- What are the signs that you're in your high vulnerability/sensitivity moment of the cycle? (It may announce itself as a feeling of being overwhelmed, intense exposure, needing to retreat, extreme reactivity to others, teariness, depression, stillness, unable to move, wanting to sleep more, acutely sensing things, having powerful dreams)
- How do you normally respond to it?
- How would you like to respond to it?
- How can you give yourself a small dose of what you want?
- Explore the concept of naming this moment as sacred time and not as a problem or weakness. How does that affect your experience of it?
- What do you discover as you engage with that space as really special rather than merely coping or blotting it out?

Session 11:
Initiation, ecstasy and shamanism

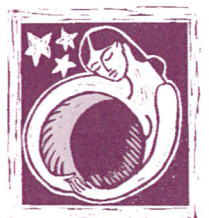

Our focus

Initiation – the process of induction into higher or deeper states of consciousness – is something that happens within a woman and not something she has to seek outside herself. It's a deeply embodied experience during her menstruating years – a psychic death and rebirth. However, if awareness of this capacity to be initiated is not understood or valued, then the opportunity is considerably weakened, if not almost lost. A woman can flip instead into times of disturbance and distress. The major points of initiation are menarche, pregnancy and birth and menopause. Yet the monthly process of the menstrual cycle and menstruation also initiates.

The cycle is the archetypal death and rebirth process. Premenstrual angst is the struggle of being undone, and menstruation an extraordinary creative tension of the Dark/Death with the epiphany of Light/Life returning. Menarche and menopause are highly amplified versions of this dynamic. And literally giving birth is an initiation like no other for death and birth are no longer just metaphorical – there is the enormous physical act of giving birth which is not without risks for both the baby and the mother even with all the support of modern medicine, the transformation of the woman into another life role, that of mother, and the ending of a former way of being.

Shamanism is a way of understanding and working with the world that takes place outside the normal consensus of reality. A shaman can access deeply altered states of consciousness to affect healing and change. Each session of this course has been a study in working with altered states, building intuitive and instinctual intelligence and learning how to integrate it into your daily life. This work has not involved any props or outer practices, only the abiding ones of attention and respect for what it is you do experience as meaningful even if it is not immediately understandable. This allows you to enter the altered states that occur naturally around menstruation. This is a form of shamanism.

Ecstasy is a key element of the work of shamanism. It's also a state that a woman can potentially access naturally at menstruation. Mircea Eliade speaks of the shaman as the professional ecstatic; amazingly in all his writings women barely get a mention except as a kind helpmeet to the man. It has taken only until recently for this to be seriously challenged. Anthropologist Barbara Tedlock writes: 'Most students of shamanism have followed Mircea Eliade in focusing their attention on masculine shamanic paths – dismemberment, evisceration and symbolic death leading to rebirth – as necessary to shamanic initiation.'[1]

Tedlock describes the foundations of the feminine path of shamanism as more spiritual and interpersonal rather than heroic and individual.[2] I would also include intimate as well. She writes that a woman on the feminine path receives her shamanic calling during menarche or pregnancy and is symbolically born into the profession.[3] I want to add that menstruation itself can be a profound opening

1 Barbara Tedlock, Ph.D., *The Woman in Shaman's Body*, Bantam Dell, New York 2005.
2 Tedlock, Barbara, *Ibid*, p.170
3 Tedlock, Barbara, *Ibid*, p.202

to calling as well. Also important is the dynamic of the menstrual cycle, the monthly round of shifting currents and moods, which develops the capacities in women for the kind of skills required for the work of shamanism. Women are matured into their profession as shaman through the monthly process of the cycle. And menstruation is quintessentially the moment for deep trance work.

In the Native American tradition men must take a sweat bath to purify themselves 'to keep their medicine effective.'[4] For women, menstruation is the means of purifying that keeps one's 'medicine effective,' a process that does not have to be struggled or sweated for, rather allowed.

While some of you may not see yourself as a shaman or even be interested in such practices you are nonetheless graced with a natural tendency for experiencing more expanded realities that are a real source of power allowing you to be much more effective in whatever field of endeavour you are involved.

[4] Muskogg Holy Man quoted in Tedlock, Barbara, *Ibid*, p.198

Menstruation was regarded as a natural time of visioning and prophecy for some indigenous peoples, such as in North America. A woman at such time could vision for her whole community. To my mind menstrual disturbances can be a nascent vision or prophecy attempting to happen that you don't yet know how to read and interpret for your community. You can also have specific visions, or a clear sense of what must be done. If women collectively were to stop 'coping with,' or medicating their distress away, but rather let the truth of it unfold, this would be a profound shamanistic act of healing for the world. I suspect there would be much we would stop putting up with. We'd say "no" more often to soul deadening and life denying practices that abound today. We'd wake up to the awful ways we are all fouling our own nest environmentally (hormonal health is also strongly connected with environmental pollution). And remember each small decision you make to do something different that says "yes" to the world is critical. So do let yourself be shaken and inspired by your symptoms into something different.

What you need to do

STEP 1: LOOK AFTER YOURSELF

Support

Get support during menstrual time and give superwoman a day off. Or as one woman suggested delegate, delegate, delegate. Can I say it any more clearly? Many menstrual tensions will bite the dust in the face of this one. And the positives of menstruation will naturally emerge.

Your ally for this month is *support*. Everyone needs it and it's not a sign of weakness but of an eminently sensible person. It's also called delegation. Cultivate this art for it's priceless in giving you the very necessary psychic space for cultivating the deep powers available through cyclical consciousness.

To help amplify the trance state, stay away from technology (in particular computers, TV and mobiles) as much as you possibly can around menstruation. This is to reduce electro magnetic radiation (EMR). You are already naturally highly charged and it's as if the EMR messes up your psychic antennae. Also avoid perfumes and strong chemicals of any kind such as chemical cleaning agents and highly perfumed shampoos. Visit your health food shop for natural products. Even avoid essential oils – although we normally think of them as good to use, emphasise your natural capacity without additives of any kind this month.

STEP 2: ASK FOR A VISION

You may be someone who has already had the experience of a prophetic dream or vision but if you haven't, ask for one this menstrual month. Ask that you be given a clear message. Remember that this prophetic dream or vision may not literally come in night dreams but as a revelation that just arises in you. Your hotspots for receiving vision are of course leading into, during and emerging out of menstruation.

STEP 3: WORK WITH TRANCE STATES

If you experience a lot of fogginess, dreaminess, or little irritating accidents just before bleeding, regard this as a period of natural trance time trying to emerge. *Slow down,* move profoundly at the pace of your body; let yourself have the dreaminess. You may notice you have a kind of 360-degree awareness, that is, you feel wide open. Revel in this expanded state. You may notice it has a prescient quality. I often used to feel I was tracking some unknown force or presence at that time and revelled in what might emerge once my focused, forceful side had taken a back seat and was no longer trying to make things happen. You can also try this when you're bleeding as it has the same effect.

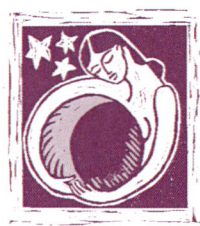

Session 12:

Time, timeliness and timing

Our focus

Timing is a great art – allowing time for things to unfold, allowing time to work on you and feeling the timeliness of things. When you work with the concept of timing and time you are recognising that there are larger forces at work than your small ego sense of the world. Those larger forces are the community or world circumstances and spiritual forces that you must cooperate with.

Timing is about sensing and trusting the ineffable forces of life; trusting one's capacity to read them. This means trusting your intuitions and feelings and, particularly, respecting your 'for no good reason' hesitations rather than labelling yourself a procrastinator. Judging yourself only digs the hole of inertia deeper and cuts you off from the intelligence at work in that hesitation. When I'm not moving on something it can be one of four things for me – I don't really want to do it and it's my being saying 'not that path;' or I'm scared and I respect that and don't bully myself (overly!); or I'm receiving information about my preparedness or rather lack of; or it simply isn't the right moment because my being somehow knows of other, as yet unknown, forces at work. So many times this last point has proved the most true for me that now, when I'm stalling, I have a degree of fascination about what might be at work and always respect it.

It's a mysterious dance of personal timing, world timing and spiritual timing. The writer, Kurt Vonnegut, once wrote that bizarre travel instructions are like dancing lessons from god. I like to regard the ups and downs of life as dancing lessons from goddess/god. Imagine you are being led somewhere, a meaning is unfolding but it requires a talent that is beyond reason to realise. The tension created when your ego is frustrated when things aren't moving the way it wants needs to be regarded as a creative opportunity for evolution rather than simply a roadblock.

The menstrual cycle reminds us that there is a time to sow and a time to reap. A time when it feels right to push for something, and a time to hold back, a time for activity and a time for rest. This notion seems somewhat quaint today when we have instant everything and we're encouraged to be switched on 24 hours a day, 7 days a week, constantly in alert mode. However it's nightmarish because it's so utterly unsustainable for our bodies and souls as well as for the planet.

The apparent limits of the rhythms of life are the very things that sustain life. Limits can indeed feel limiting in the moment. However limits provide the crucible or container in which your ego has to face something. Understandably, your ego doesn't like this moment of being pulled in or stopped. A limit will always momentarily feel like you are personally being thwarted and who really likes not getting their own way. But rather like a child who needs boundaries to develop well, so your ego needs the container of limits to mature – the maturity, in particular, to recognise the interconnection and interdependence of all life. Rather like the irritation of the grit in the oyster shell that helps create the pearl, the 'irritation' of the limit becomes the opening to something wholly new and richer.

What you need to do

STEP 1: LOOK AFTER YOURSELF

Focus on the ally *serenity* this month. This quality will allow a certain equanimity with what is and allow you to 'feel' the World more, to feel the larger currents at work that are important to work with. And let your way of caring for the power of menstruation come spontaneously this month.

With regard to diet and other health practices, what do you feel you need to improve this month? Go ahead and do that.

> ### Serenity
> *Cruise, glide, keep a certain detachment from the stuff of the world, even if it looks momentarily about to collapse, maintain a certain serene bubble of detachment about you.*

STEP 2: FOLLOW YOUR INNER TIDES

During the whole of this month, respect the times when you pull back or hesitate. Be curious and respect the hesitation rather than chastising yourself for not acting. Accept your tendencies and see what happens. Think of these hesitations as a kind of knowing at work. I realise that sometimes it's important to push yourself also. To 'feel the fear and do it anyway,' as Susan Jeffers says in her book of the same name. But we also need another book called 'Feel the fear and don't do it because it's possible something much more interesting is trying to unfold for which you don't have the full information yet and you could go off half cocked' (although I'm not sure the book trade would go at such long title). Appreciate your moods and energy levels during the cycle. If you feel seized to do something, do it. Equally, if you feel the tide turning and pulling in, don't force anything, just take pleasure in it.

> ### *Reflect on your experience of this in your journal:*
> - Was it easy to do? Were you still judging yourself?
> - What were you confronted with? What opened up?
> - How do you feel about yourself now?
> - Did you have a small sense of timing or timeliness?
> - What are you noticing about this course over time? How has the steady progress of time and attention affected your experience of yourself and your goals?

Session 13:

Embodying your wisdom

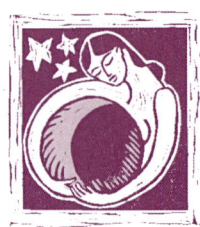

Our focus

The menstrual cycle is your wisdom growing process, a means of restoring you to a larger consciousness, to a deep sense of oneness with the World. Robert Sardello speaks of midlife crisis as the world seeking to become conscious in us, of becoming 'the world's awareness rather than individuals who are aware of the world based upon our needs and desires.'[1] This same dynamic is happening at menstruation as well – a kind of homeopathic dose of World awareness each month, a process that is heightened many fold over at menopause. This is wisdom at work.

The work of rhythm provides your passage into this consciousness. It's this very movement of expansion and contraction, of assertion and hesitation, of our ego going out to meet the world and then getting undone that knits together the World and you. Starhawk, the feminist activist and spiritual teacher, reminds us that 'Life expands; death imposes limitations. When the two forces are in balance a rich diversity of life forms can co-exist.'[2] This is wisdom.

Wisdom is also the Deep Feminine presence. She is known as you engage with the world rather than try to control it. As you are touched, this presence is known. As you let yourself be 'worked on' by the vicissitudes of life and allow yourself to be changed She has the means of manifesting. As you allow yourself to be opened She is known. Exquisite intimacy is Her song. However, the announcement of Her presence can feel like chaos and trouble. We often equate the feminine, and women for that matter, with just that. Neither women nor the feminine are chaos or trouble. Rather it *feels* chaotic for the ego to let go of control – to handle an Unknown presence that it cannot control, neatly package and commodify. The chaos is a signal of the potential emergence of Her presence, so hang in there.

The reintegration of the repressed feminine is going to take some struggle, a willingness to be stripped bare and experience a sacrifice. A threshold has to be crossed that requires an enormous courage and 'an act of unflinching self-discernment.'[3] That threshold is crossed monthly for women as you experience the premenstrual ego death and have your showdown with the critic. It is amplified many fold over as a woman crosses the menopause. As you face that critical force in yourself, as you are willing to let yourself be undone so you have the means of building 'unflinching self-discernment.' This self-discernment is your ally for fully embodying your power and wisdom.

You come to a place where the world is inside you now, you are rooted in something so much bigger and greater than yourself that is a source of inspiration and guidance. You can act cleanly, with wisdom and grace, have little concern for other's opinions, hold your own counsel yet can deeply listen and value the other, and are not easily seduced or charmed.

[1] Sardello, Robert, *Love and the World,* Lindisfarne Books 2001 Great Barrington, MA, p.33

[2] Starhawk, *Dreaming the Dark,* Unwin Hyman Ltd London 1990, p.38

[3] Tarnas, Richard, *The Passion of the Western Mind,* Ballantine Books, New York, 1991, p.444

How did you get to this place? Through living, loving, engaging, observing, and going the round each month into the underworld, and not feeling ashamed to be stripped bare and challenged.

As you enter the underworld you face the dark side of the Feminine, the death dealing side. If you want to understand the Feminine you have to understand her, the force of destruction. To wrestle with her is to be hung out on meat hooks to dry, to be shot through with a thousand holes, to be so wrung out as to be a lifeless rag doll. Take it as a compliment, she's got big business for you and she wants someone who has lived into the deepest darkest corners of herself and claimed every millimetre of her being. Only then may you be able to claim the authority of the Feminine, but not before. So each month, as you face the harshness of your inner critic, think of it as a kind of spiritual practice, such as sitting in meditation or praying. It's a tad tougher but your goal is the honing of this self-discernment that gives entry to the sanctum of the Feminine.

We probably need about 30 years of menstruating, going the round each month, coming up battle scarred – sometimes losing, sometimes winning, or maybe negotiating a uneasy truce. But in this round a priceless understanding is forged that allows us to harvest something quite sacred and blessed at menstruation itself, an experience that we might come to know continuously in our lives. It gives us the capacity to handle the creative tensions of life. It's called wisdom. There are no short cuts to this knowing – it's the potential gift that your body offers you each month as you bleed.

What you need to do

STEP 1: LOOK AFTER YOURSELF

Self-interest is your ally this month. Self-interest is you tending to your own needs. Sometimes this can feel like you have to go against others' needs. It's inevitable and how to deal with competing needs is the stuff of relationship life. For those of you who are mothers and who struggle with claiming time for yourself often thinking that it's selfish, remember this act of self-care is also an act of care for your children. To abandon your own needs serves nobody least of all your children. The more you can assert your own needs and ideas, the stronger the inner vessel of your being becomes and the more effective you are in the world and the more capacity you have to really be there for others.

Self-interest

Practice undiluted self-interest. And no, it's not selfishness; it's self-interestedness and self-preservation. Others indeed may not like it but, remember, that could be their own apparent selfishness speaking. This is truly the time when you unashamedly give to yourself.

Environmental pollution has an enormous impact on our wellbeing. To minimise its effects in our personal lives means taking actions that help the world as well. Here are a few ideas for your health:

- Use green cleaning products.
- Keep soft plastic out of your life as much as possible including plastic bags, cling film, bubble wrap.
- Avoid aerosols and propellant sprays of any kind.
- Stop and think before you pile on skin care products – they're made from a toxic cocktail of chemicals. There are products available now that are made from natural ingredients, although you still need to be wary of some of these. Read labels assiduously and minimise use as much as possible.
- Avoid petrochemical based pesticides in your garden.
- Radically reduce mobile phone use, or, best of all, avoid using them altogether except for emergencies.
- Eat organically and biodynamically produced food and avoid genetically modified and irradiated food.

 Check out *The Wild Genie: The Healing Power of Menstruation* or *Walking with Genie: The Modern Woman's Menstrual Health Guide* by Alexandra Pope, for a list of more suggestions.
www.wildgenie.com

STEP 2: GATHER YOUR WISDOM

Think of serving the world as a daily act. Some days you'll probably feel you're better at it than others. It's both about what you do *and* who you are, the quality of the way you act and be. Some of you may be drawn to grand projects, others seemingly more mundane, more intimate and quiet ones; some go for more practical, others more ineffable. However seemingly grand the act, no act is grander than another – they are all needed. You can serve the world by simply smiling at another being, connecting with your neighbour, including your plant and animal neighbours.

In particular, think about what your strengths are that you can offer. Name them out loud then write them in your journal.

When you menstruate this month, actively think of yourself and the World as one. Feel the intimacy with the Greater Whole and your responsibility towards it. And above all feel how you are spoken to, what you are called to attend to for the World's sake. What lights you up is always a sure guide.

STEP 3: RELISH THE JOURNEY

Reflect on and relish the journey that you have been on over the past 13 sessions:

- How connected do you feel to the cycle and to yourself?
- What discoveries have you made about yourself? How do you feel within yourself?
- Do you feel intimations of Wisdom maturing in you? What are you noticing in yourself that speaks to you of that?
- If you were to rate your acceptance of yourself compared with the beginning of the course, has it changed?
- How has your calling spoken to you, and how well do you feel you are following it?
- How do your experiences at menstruation speak to you of the World? What might the World be speaking through you?
- Check out the intentions and goals you had at the beginning of the course. Have you reached any of your goals? How have things changed?
- What have you got out of the course?

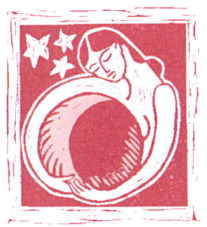

Epilogue:
Women are blessed

Women are blessed.

The menstrual cycle is our inner guidance system, initiating us into and anointing us with ever deepening revelation and wisdom.

The movements of the cycle are like the breath catching, like the snagging of threads in a garment. A sudden shift in gear, a cloud scudding across the sun, a small irritation, a distraction. Quiet, subtle, demanding your attention. Tripping you into different realities, perspectives and understandings. Breaking the mould of the cultural mindset. Stopping you from becoming an endless doing machine. Reminding you of yourself and making you sensitive to the World.

It's the crucible in which you can forge internal authority. Attention to and acceptance of the conditions of the cycle cultivate that authority. Constant resistance or denial of the life of the body will lock you into an in-between world: a perpetual adolescence of the spirit, an unripened emotional life.

If you know how to let go in to the high sensitivity of the menstrual world you have an amazing opening to greater intimacy and emotional maturity, to wisdom and altered states.

This is your power. An embodied power, richly woven out of the strands of a woman's deep engagement with both inner and outer worlds. It emanates from your willingness to hold to yourself in dark and challenging moments. A mix of heart and head, instinct and intellect. Most of all this power comes from your capacity to surrender. In that moment you can truly touch the awesome presence of the Feminine.[1]

---

[1] Adapted from: Pope, Alexandra, 'Celebrating the Genie' in *The Wild Genie: The Healing Power of Menstruation,* Sally Milner Publishing, Bowral, 2001, p.220

FINAL NOTE

I hope you have found this journey into the power of the menstrual cycle and menstruation fruitful and vivifying; that you are enjoying a new and stronger relationship with yourself that feels kinder, more empowering and affirming of female ways; that you are using your power in the world more effectively and feeling a stronger sense of connection and calling to the World. And for those of you who suffer with menstrual problems that you are experiencing the wisdom of menstruation easing and healing your symptoms.

With warmest blessings

Alexandra

PS: I'd love to hear how you've gone with the Quest. Please send any feedback to:
info@womensquest.org

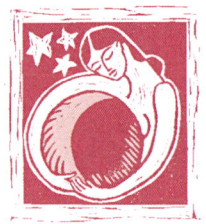

Appendix:
Menarche Ritual

A highly significant rite of passage, menarche, your very first period, is the initiatory moment into the depths of yourself as a woman – the beginning of a journey of spiritual initiation that culminates at menopause. Menarche is your first set of instructions in the mystery school of the deep feminine. It is critical that this time be recognised and anointed.

Amongst some of the indigenous people of North America it was believed that any significant dream or dreams that occur at the time of the first period gave insights into the future of the girl – it would hold some vision for her life. Just as a boy must go on a vision quest in nature to get his sacred dream for his life so the dream that accompanies a girl's first bleeding is her sacred guidance. I also believe that at each menstruation one can ignite that visionary capacity.

However today, obscured by our mechanistic worldview that sees the body as an assemblage of physiological processes, menarche and subsequently menstruation have become devoid of all spirit and soul. Our literalist and mechanistic worldview have sapped us of our ability to see hidden depths, losing our shamanic capacities to live within multiple realities. Asleep to menarche's significance we pass over this opening, treating it as *just* a biological marker of a girl growing up.

If the cycle is a basic template that helps to create the Ground of a woman's being, missing the doorway to it at menarche is to undermine something enormously significant at the core of a woman. How you cross this threshold will influence your sense of self, your relationship to your body, your experience of menstruation and sexuality, the processes of pregnancy and birth, your relationship to others, your power and expression in the world and capacity to trust life.

RECOVERING YOUR OWN MENARCHE

For those of you whose experience of menarche was neither positive nor celebrated all is not lost. It is possible through ritual enactment to recover this moment and re-configure it for yourself. There are two stages to this. First you need to recollect your actual experience and consider how you would have liked it to be. Then create a menarche ritual for yourself. In the days leading up to and after the ritual, pay attention to your dreams, you might have a significant 'menarche' dream.

Stage 1.
Recollecting the past

Remember back to the time of your first period and allow as much detail as possible to surface. Write freely. Here are some questions to get you going:[1]

- How old were you when you had your first period?
- Where were you when you first saw the blood? And what was your initial reaction?
- How did it feel physically and emotionally?
- Who was the first person you told and what was their response?
- Were you prepared and if so how was that done and by whom? (Some girls learnt informally through their sisters or friends in the schoolyard)
- What were some of the messages, spoken and unspoken, positive and negative, you received about menstruation and becoming a woman?
- What was the response of your parents/guardian and other family members?
- What kind of response did you get from friends? Did your relationship change in any way with those who weren't yet menstruating?
- Did your relationship with any of the family change?
- What was your mother's experience of menstruation? Your aunts'? Your grandmothers'?
- Did you have any kind of celebration?
- What was the school's approach to menstruation and the needs of menstruating girls?
- What would you have liked to have heard and didn't from your mother? From your father?
- Did you change in your relationship to the world and in your sense of self after menstruation began? What became important to you?
- Did you have any significant dream or recurring dreams around menarche?
- What are the personal messages you tell yourself today about menstruation?
- Do you notice any similarities in your current attitude to and experience of menstruation and your early experiences of it?

[1] A number of the questions are taken from **Jane Bennett's** *A Blessing Not a Curse*, Sally Milner Publishing 2002, p.56

Stage 2. Creating your Ritual

Ideally this needs to be done with at least one other person; however, if there is no one with whom you can comfortably do this ceremony you can do it on your own. Let the ritual grow inside you over a period of time. Set the idea for it and give yourself a week or two or three to feel and dream into it – how you would like it to be, the most auspicious time to do it. I tended to do rituals when I was bleeding, but it might be significant to do it on the dark of the moon or as the new moon is just appearing in the sky.

MENARCHE RITUAL FOR TWO OR MORE

The following is a simple process. Feel free to add your own embellishments. If you're doing it on your own you will need to play both roles as I describe them below. Or you can right a letter to Mum, the Great Goddess, or whoever feels appropriate, to release the old story and then write another, this time to your young self telling her about this amazing journey she is about to embark on and whatever else you would like her to know about herself.

Allow time. Put aside at least a whole evening if there are two of you. With more people it might require the best part of a day.

Create an altar. Include a photo of yourself around the age of the first bleed, or some symbol of that young girl, along with any other sacred or special objects you have that feel appropriate. It might be important to have symbols of the women in your family such as photos and/or mementoes of your mother, grandmothers, great grandmothers, aunts and sisters, or significant carers in your life. You might also want to add some flowers and candles. Make it feel special and beautiful to you.

Tell the story:

1. Tell the story of your experience of menarche – the good, the bad and the ugly – to your ritual partner. Let it all come out. Take as long as you need. The partner's task is to listen deeply as you tell the story.

2. Now draw an imaginary circle and step into it. This time tell the story from that circle as though you are that younger self finding your menstrual blood for the first time. Tell the story in the present tense.

3. Step out of the circle and tell your partner what you would have liked, what you needed to hear but didn't. This might include the acknowledgement of budding talents, strengths, attributes or inner qualities, so that something singular and special about you is seen and named.

Blessing. Step back into the imaginary magic circle and become your younger self again. Your partner is now going to be proxy for Mum/Dad/parental guardian. You can decide who you want her to be – it can be more than one person. Your partner now speaks back to you the words you needed to hear at menarche, but didn't, in a strong, clear and declarative voice. She will 'see' in you and name those talents and strengths. Beforehand you might decide whether you want the partner to also add her own positive observations.

Receive her words. Take your time to drink it all in, take it deeply into your being.

Gifts. You can include simple gifts at this point. I think simple, yet, symbolic, is important. One flower might be all that's needed – a flower still in bud form that will blossom in the ensuing days. Or a piece of jewellery you have bought for yourself specially to mark this occasion. Have your partner give you the gift.

Create: Draw an image, write a poem or any words to hold and celebrate this moment if you feel drawn to.

Final words: Is there is anything more that needs to be spoken? If not, you can close the ceremony with a thank you to your partner.

Change roles. Your ritual partner may go through the process if she so chooses.

Feast. To finish the ritual you might enjoy a celebratory drink and/or meal together.

Menstrual Dreaming Chart

On the first day of your period you can start recording your thoughts and feelings on day one of the Menstrual Dreaming Chart. Watch the patterns of your cycles unfold as you continue to record over a number of months.

Begin a new chart at the start of each period. Blank sheets suitable for colour or black and white copying are included on the next two pages.

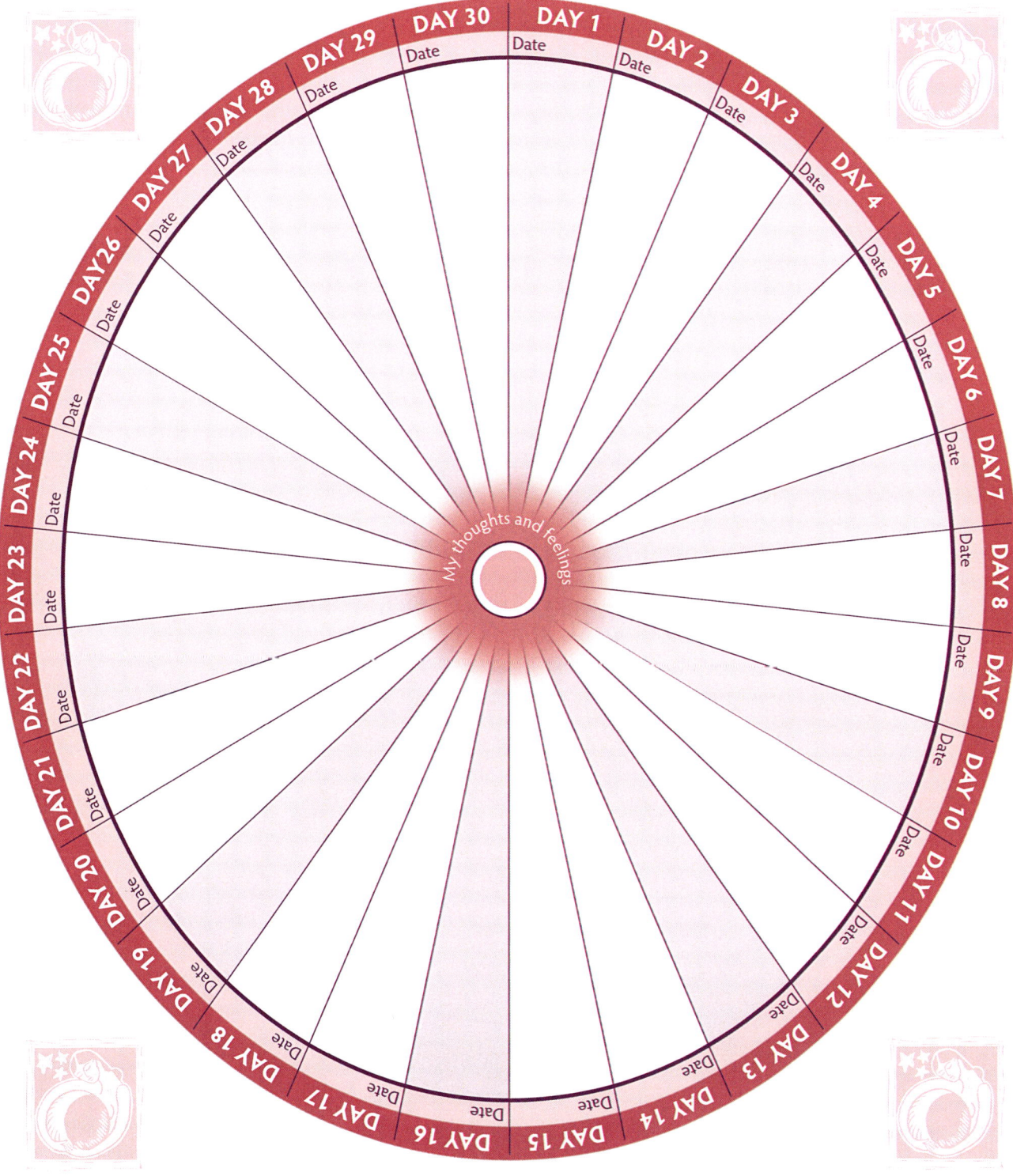

© Alexandra Pope 2006

Menstrual Dreaming Chart

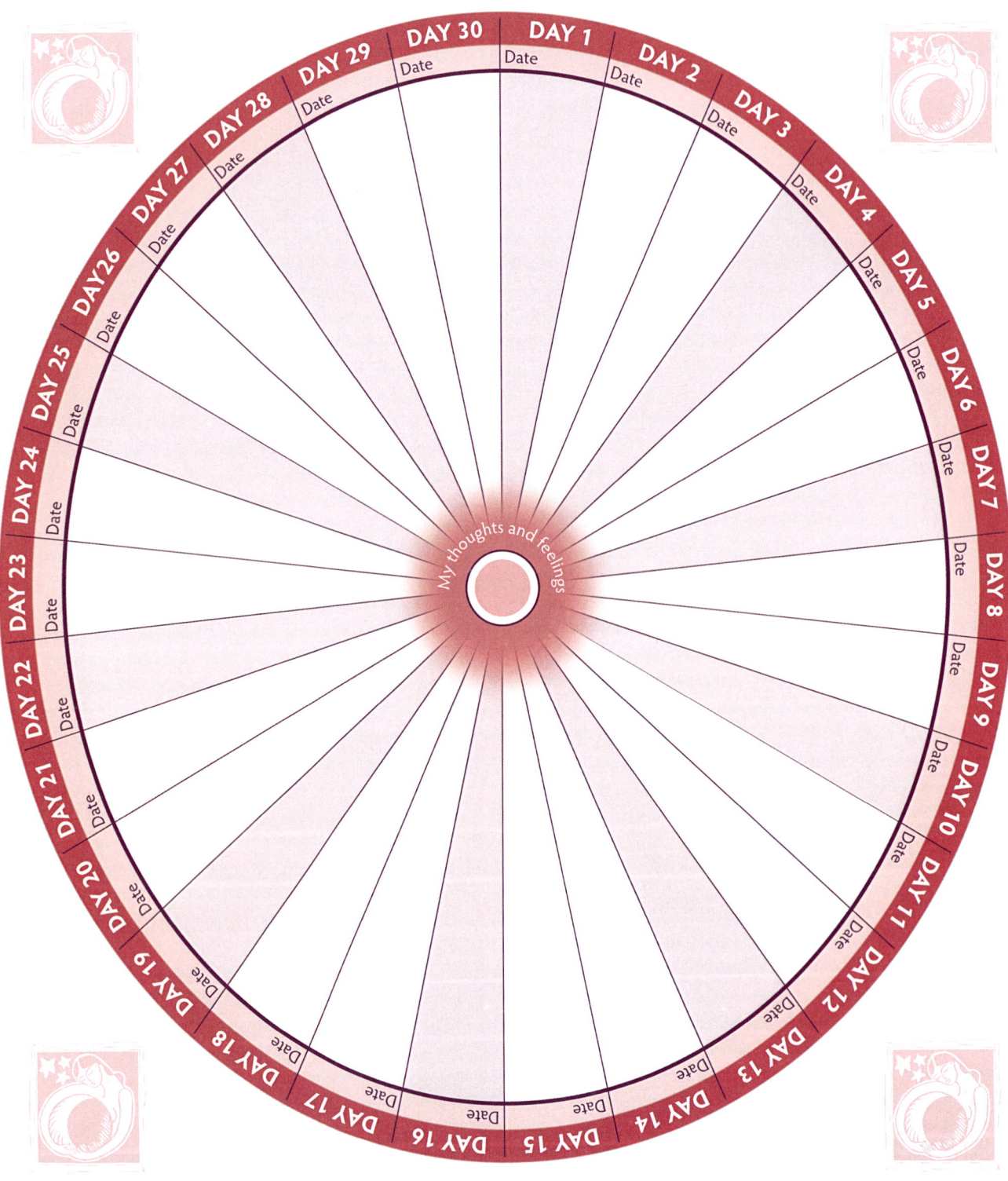

Menstrual Dreaming Chart

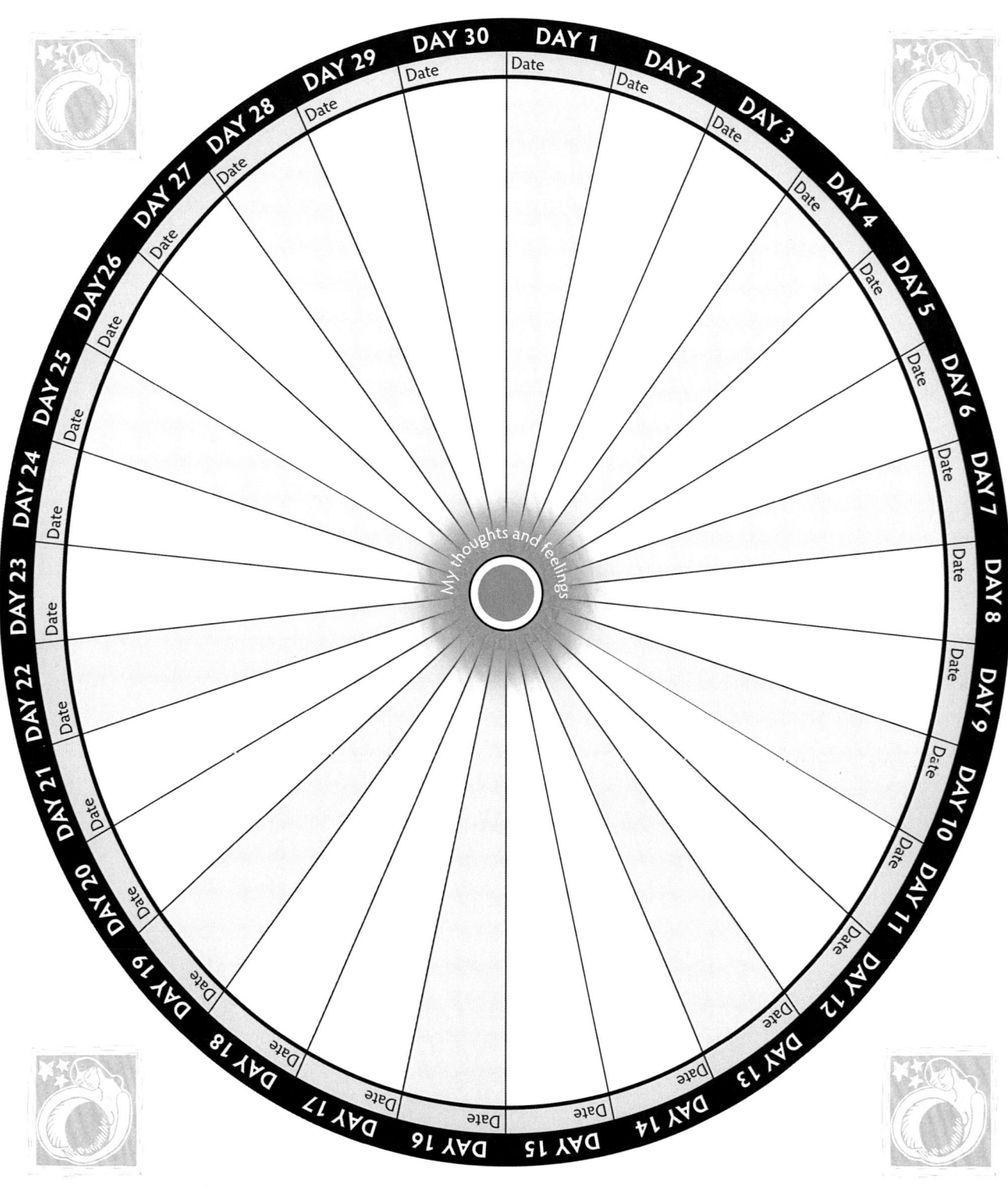

ACKNOWLEDGEMENTS

A big thank you to:

Amy Scully for your wonderful support of this work and your original ideas and insightful feedback;

Jane Bennett, Julee Cunningham, Jen Fox, Maree Lipschitz, Fran Montague and Shushann Movsessian for the various ways you cared for this text and my work in general;

Patricia Hoyle for your thoughtful editing as always,

and to Toni Lumsden for the beautiful design.

I am very grateful.

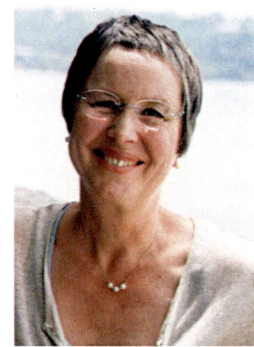

With over 20 years experience as a psychotherapist, Alexandra is author of **The Wild Genie: The Healing Power of Menstruation** *(Sally Milner Publishing, 2001)*, and co-author of **The Pill: are you sure it's for you** *(Allen and Unwin, 2008)*.

She has pioneered a new approach to women's psychological and spiritual development based on the power of the cycle. She now works as a facilitator, coach and healer in UK and Europe offering programmes for women based on her work.

For more information on Alexandra's workshops, books, coaching and counselling:

website: www.womensquest.org
email: info@womensquest.org